MOTIVATIONAL INTERVIEWING IN HEALTH CARE

Applications of Motivational Interviewing

Stephen Rollnick and William R. Miller, *Series Editors*

Since the publication of Miller and Rollnick's classic *Motivational Interviewing*, MI has become hugely popular as a tool for facilitating many different kinds of positive behavior change. This highly practical series demonstrates MI approaches for a range of applied contexts and with a variety of populations. Each accessible volume reviews the empirical evidence base and presents easy-to-implement strategies, illuminating concrete examples, and clear-cut guidance on integrating MI with other interventions.

Motivational Interviewing in the Treatment of Psychological Problems
Hal Arkowitz, Henny A. Westra, William R. Miller, and Stephen Rollnick, Editors

Motivational Interviewing in Health Care: Helping Patients Change Behavior
Stephen Rollnick, William R. Miller, and Christopher C. Butler

MOTIVATIONAL INTERVIEWING IN HEALTH CARE

Helping Patients Change Behavior

Stephen Rollnick
William R. Miller
Christopher C. Butler

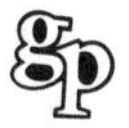

THE GUILFORD PRESS
New York London

A Division of Guilford Publications, Inc.
72 Spring Street, New York, NY 10012
www.guilford.com

Printed in the United States of America

This book is printed on acid-free paper.

Last digit is print number: 9 8 7 6 5

Library of Congress Cataloging-in-Publication Data

Rollnick, Stephen, 1952–
Motivational interviewing in health care : helping patients change behavior / by Stephen Rollnick, William R. Miller, Christopher C. Butler.
p. ; cm. — (Applications of motivational interviewing)
Includes bibliographical references and index.
ISBN-13: 978-1-59385-613-7 (hardcover : alk. paper)
ISBN-10: 1-59385-613-X (hardcover : alk. paper)
ISBN-13: 978-1-59385-612-0 (pbk. : alk. paper)
ISBN-10: 1-59385-612-1 (pbk. : alk. paper)
1. Health counseling. 2. Motivational interviewing. 3. Health behavior. 4. Behavior modification. I. Miller, William R. II. Butler, Christopher, 1959– III. Title. IV. Series.
[DNLM: 1. Behavior Therapy—methods. 2. Interview, Psychological. 3. Motivation. WM 425 R754m 2008]
R727.4.R65 2008
362.1'04256—dc22

2007020536

To my dear father, Julian. Thank you for many things,
including your lucid advice and support
in the writing of this book. —S. R.

To my son, Jayson. May I always be for you
the same loving, guiding presence
with which my parents blessed me. —W. R. M.

To Judith and our children,
Caitlin, Eva, and Charles, who helped me
so much to find a way. —C. C. B.

About the Authors

Stephen Rollnick, PhD, is a clinical psychologist and Professor of Health Care Communication in the Department of Primary Care and Public Health at Cardiff University, Wales, United Kingdom. He practiced in a primary care setting for 16 years and then became a teacher and researcher on the subject of communication. Dr. Rollnick has written books on motivational interviewing and health behavior change and has a special interest in challenging consultations in health and social care. He has published widely in scientific journals and has taught practitioners and trainers in many countries throughout the world.

William R. Miller, PhD, is Emeritus Distinguished Professor of Psychology and Psychiatry at the University of New Mexico, where he joined the faculty in 1976. He served as Director of Clinical Training for UNM's American Psychological Association-approved doctoral program in clinical psychology and as Codirector of UNM's Center on Alcoholism, Substance Abuse, and Addictions (CASAA). Dr. Miller's publications include 35 books and more than 400 articles and chapters. He introduced the concept of motivational interviewing in a 1983 article. The Institute for Scientific Information names him as one of the world's most cited scientists.

Christopher C. Butler, MD, is Professor of Primary Care Medicine and head of the Department of Primary Care and Public Health at Cardiff University. He trained in medicine at the University of Cape Town and in clinical epidemiology at the University of Toronto. For his doctoral work, under the direction of Stephen Rollnick, he developed and evaluated behavior change counseling and conducted qualitative research into patients' perceptions of advice against smoking from clinicians. Dr. Butler has published more than 70 papers, mainly on health behavior change and common infections. He has a general medical practice in a former coal-mining town in south Wales.

Preface

This book is for any health care practitioner who spends time encouraging patients to consider behavior change. The list is quite a long one: nurses, doctors, dieticians, psychologists, counselors, health educators, dentists, dental hygienists, social workers, physical and occupational therapists, podiatrists, and sometimes even people who answer the office telephones. The list of behaviors that might need to be changed is also long: smoking, diet, exercise, medication changes, alcohol consumption, fluid intake, the learning of new procedures, use of new aids, uptake of services, and so on.

It was health care practitioners who brought the potential for motivational interviewing in health settings to our attention. Each day they see patients whose health could be greatly improved by behavior change. Usually, their patients are not asking for help with this. The practitioners do their best to encourage, persuade, cajole, counsel, or advise their patients to make changes. They have seldom received training and preparation in how to promote health behavior change, and often have only a few minutes per patient to do so in the face of many other competing clinical imperatives. We have listened to the problems, frustrations, and practical constraints of frontline health care practitioners:

"I tell them and tell them what to do, but they won't do it."
"It's my job just to give them the facts, and that's all I can do."
"These people lead very difficult lives, and I understand why they smoke."
"I'm not a counselor; I diagnose and manage medical conditions."
"Some of my patients are in complete denial."

We found that passion (and compassion) ran high about patient predicaments and how best to respond to them.

When we first wrote about motivational interviewing we had counselors in mind, and we focused on patient problems with alcohol and other drugs. These patients had tough behavior change problems and their lives frequently lay in ruins. Despite the devastating consequences of their drinking or drug use, their ambivalence about change was striking. We quickly learned that lecturing, arguing, and warning did not work well with ambivalent people, and over time we developed the more gentle approach that would come to be called motivational interviewing. The focus was on helping these people talk about and resolve their ambivalence about behavior change, using their own motivation, energy, and commitment to do it.

Soon after publication of the first edition of *Motivational Interviewing* (Miller & Rollnick, 1991), it became apparent to us and others that this method could be useful outside the addiction field. Indeed, struggles with ambivalence about change are not at all unique to addictions, but are characteristic of being human. Presently, much of health care involves helping patients to manage long-term conditions where outcomes can be greatly influenced by lifestyle behavior change. Yet patients often resist well-intentioned efforts to persuade them into change. There are certainly limits to what a practitioner can do, but there is also great potential for change. Certainly, motivation to change is better elicited than imposed. Humane, respectful, and effective conversations about behavior change clearly have a place in many health care settings.

Within a few years, publications were appearing on the use of motivational interviewing in managing hypertension, diabetes, obesity, heart disease, medication adherence, and a range of psychiatric and psychological problems. There are now over 160 randomized clinical trials of motivational interviewing, with publications on the method doubling every 3 years (see *www.motivationalinterview.org*).

We have now taught motivational interviewing to a diverse range of practitioners. It is being used by providers in family practice, cardiac and cognitive rehabilitation, renal medicine, diabetes care, physical therapy, fitness coaching, dental care, mental health counseling, vocal/speech therapy, and public health education. The challenge for us has been to find a way for health care practitioners to use elements of motivational interviewing in the "hurly-burly" of everyday clinical practice.

A first step in this direction was a book called *Health Behavior Change* (Rollnick, Mason, & Butler, 1999). Cautious about diluting and simplifying motivational interviewing beyond recognition, we all but avoided any reference to it. The book merely described some useful, practical strategies, many of them developed in health care settings that adhered to the essential *spirit* of motivational interviewing—using good rapport to help the patient explore and resolve ambivalence about change.

Teams of researchers followed a similar path, developing and testing a variety of adaptations of motivational interviewing that spanned many settings and problem areas. By the time the second edition of *Motivational Interviewing* (Miller & Rollnick, 2002) was published, adaptations had emerged with names such as brief negotiation, behavior change counseling, a behavior "check-up," and brief motivational interviewing. Behind them all was the same idea about evoking patients' own motivations for change.

This book is a new synthesis on how to bring the heart of motivational interviewing into everyday health care practice. Few practitioners have the time, need, or inclination to become counselors. Our goal here is to convey just enough of the essential method of motivational interviewing to make it accessible, learnable, useful, and effective in health care practice.

We have tried to capture the essence of the approach without resorting to foreign-sounding technical jargon. In this book we use the metaphor of a guide. We suggest that a guiding style is something used naturally in everyday life to help other people, particularly with changing their behavior or learning new skills. We contrast it with two other everyday communication styles: directing and following. Directing has come to predominate in health care practice, precisely as it did in addiction treatment during the 1970s and 1980s, and with the same predictable problems and limitations. The art of skillful guiding is all too often lost in the hectic pace of modern health care. Some think that there is no longer time for it in health care. But we believe that when time is short and behavior change is vital, a guiding style is most likely to efficiently produce better outcomes for patients and practitioners alike.

From this simple starting point come a number of implications for training and practice. *Motivational interviewing is a refined form of the familiar process of guiding.* The skillful practitioner is someone who can shift flexibly among directing, guiding, and following styles in response to patients' needs. In other words, motivational interviewing does not displace, but rather complements, the communication skills you have already developed.

This method is something that you can continue to learn and refine throughout a lifetime of practice. This is so precisely because you can learn it from your patients. Once you know what to listen for, every patient consultation becomes a source of learning and gives you feedback about how you're doing. When you finish reading this book, you won't be proficient in this guiding style of motivational interviewing. Instead, if we have written well, you will know how to learn it from your own patients.

In Part I we begin by offering an overview of motivational interviewing, its evidence base, and how it fits within the broader context of health care. We then describe the three communication styles of directing, guiding, and following, and present three specific core skills: asking, informing, and listening. In Part II we show how these skills can be refined and used in the service of the guiding style of motivational interviewing. Finally, in Part III we offer some practical examples and guidelines for improving your comfort and skill in using motivational interviewing in practice. A final chapter looks beyond the individual consultation to how the service environment might also enhance health behavior change.

STEPHEN ROLLNICK, PHD
WILLIAM R. MILLER, PHD
CHRISTOPHER C. BUTLER, MD

REFERENCES

Miller, W. R., & Rollnick, S. (1991). *Motivational interviewing: Preparing people to change addictive behavior.* New York: Guilford Press.

Miller, W. R., & Rollnick, S. (2002). *Motivational interviewing (2nd ed.): Preparing people for change.* New York: Guilford Press.

Rollnick, S., Mason, P., & Butler, C. (1999). *Health behavior change: A guide for practitioners.* Edinburgh, UK: Churchill Livingstone.

Acknowledgments

We acknowledge with heartfelt thanks the contributions of practitioners we have met in training, too many to mention, who helped us clarify our thinking and understanding.

The inspiration and suggestions from colleagues in MINT, the Motivational Interviewing Network of Trainers (*www.motivationalinterview.org*), were a regular source of support. It was typical of this group to shower us with ideas when we put questions to them in meetings and on the electronic mailing list that connects us in lively discussion. Jeff Allison and Gary Rose helped us to clarify, in training efforts and through discussion, the content and boundaries of the three-styles framework. Feedback and suggestions from Tom Barth and Pip Mason enriched the material on aspirations for behavior change in Chapter 10. Bob Mash and colleagues from the South African MISA (Motivational Interviewing in South Africa) trainers' group provided stories, vignettes, and suggestions that were used to construct case studies and accounts of consultations and services in the HIV/AIDS field. Colleagues from PATA (Pediatric AIDS Treatment in Africa), particularly Dr. Paul Roux, provided countless examples of the triumph of hope, commitment, and creativity in the face of adversity. Ralf Demmel fed us with papers on parental scaffolding; Michael Robling gave his time and experience to discussions about diabetes care; and Claire Lane, Linda Speck, and Adrienne Cook gave us feedback about cardiac rehabilitation and lucid accounts of their efforts to change the culture of services. Peter Prescott and Carolina Yahne wrote to us on more than one occasion about the principle and practice of conveying hope. Conversations with Valerie

Dougall in the software design world helped enormously in considering how ideas can be made accessible to learners. We also thank Carrie McCorkindale, Barbara B. Walker, Anne E. Kazak, and Sheila K. Stevens for their help in reviewing an earlier draft of the manuscript.

Our families helped us in more ways than one. We thank our partners, Sheila, Kathy, and Judith, for supporting our writing efforts, and Jacob Rollnick for highlighting the role of high emotion in motivational interviewing when helping others to change at home (no names mentioned). Julian Rollnick scrutinized every word and offered invaluable advice and encouragement. Finally, we thank our editors at The Guilford Press, Jim Nageotte and Barbara Watkins, for their truly expert help in shaping the structure and content of this book.

Contents

PART I. BEHAVIOR CHANGE AND MOTIVATIONAL INTERVIEWING

1 Motivational Interviewing: Principles and Evidence 3

2 How Motivational Interviewing Fits into Health Care Practice 11

PART II. CORE SKILLS OF MOTIVATIONAL INTERVIEWING

3 Practicing Motivational Interviewing 33

4 Asking 44

5 Listening 65

6 Informing 86

PART III. PUTTING IT ALL TOGETHER

7 Integrating the Skills 111

8 Case Examples of a Guiding Style 121

9 Getting Better at Guiding 140

10 Beyond the Consultation 157

Epilogue: Some Maps to Guide You 173

Appendix A. Learning More about Motivational Interviewing 177

Appendix B. A Topical Bibliography of Research on Motivational Interviewing 183

Index 205

PART I

BEHAVIOR CHANGE AND MOTIVATIONAL INTERVIEWING

CHAPTER 1

Motivational Interviewing

Principles and Evidence

During the 20th century remarkable advances occurred in curing acute illnesses. The successful treatment and control of infectious diseases significantly prolonged life expectancy. Traumatic injuries that were once fatal or permanently disabling are now treatable. Some forms of organ failure can be addressed through dialysis, transplantation, and bypass surgery. From the perspective of health care capabilities, populations in developed nations should be healthier than ever before.

Yet there are signs that today's young adults may be the first generation in modern history to be less healthy than their parents. Respiratory diseases and cancers, diabetes and obesity, heart and liver disease, and some psychological problems, such as depression, are all strongly linked to health behavior and lifestyle. A majority of the maladies that now cause people to consult health care professionals (e.g., physicians, dentists, nurses, chiropractors) are largely preventable or remediable through health behavior change.

In the developing world, and in the underbelly of large cities everywhere, people in inadequate living conditions also struggle against a level of adversity that threatens their health. They consult health care practitioners in difficult circumstances in which a similar range of health behavior concerns arise, and they often feel that their health is not necessarily something they can control. Yet here, too, behavior change is a key component of many risks to health, from smoking, excessive alcohol use, and poor diet to water purification, infant feeding practices, and the prevention of infectious diseases.

In the 21st century, health care is increasingly about long-term condition management and thus about health behavior change—those things that people can do to improve their health. And so it is hard to think of a health care setting or professional role, a clinical diagnosis or a health care problem, in which patient behavior change is not a potentially important contributor to prevention, to treatment, or to the maintenance of health. However, most people who seek health care still seem to be looking for a medical cure. They expect the practitioner to ask a series of questions and then prescribe a treatment that will restore them to health or, at least, alleviate their symptoms. In other words, no matter how they may mistreat themselves, the responsibility for curing them is seen to lie with the physician, the nurse, or the overall health care system.

In the 21st century, health care is increasingly about long-term condition management and thus about health behavior change—those things that people can do to improve their health.

If you are a doctor, nurse, physical therapist, health social worker, dentist, dental hygienist, dietician, podiatrist, counselor, health psychologist, or other health care professional, you probably have many conversations about behavior change in the course of your typical work day. What is often less clear is how a practitioner should approach this topic. Should you:

Explain what patients could do differently in the interest of their health?
Advise and persuade them to change their behavior?
Warn them what will happen if they don't change their ways?
Take time to counsel them about *how* to change their behavior?
Refer them to a specialist?

This book was written to help you have productive conversations with patients about behavior change. In particular, we describe a gentle form of counseling known as motivational interviewing (MI), which has been found effective in fostering change across a wide range of health behaviors.

The clinical method of MI, first described in 1983, was initially developed as a brief intervention for problem drinking, in which patient motivation is a common obstacle to change. Starting in the 1990s, MI began to be tested with other health problems, particularly chronic diseases, in which behavior change is key and patient motivation is a common challenge. There have been positive trials of MI in the management of cardiovascular disease, diabetes, diet, hypertension, psychosis, and pathological gambling and in the treatment and prevention of HIV infection. Clinical trials of MI have been published across a broad range of behavior-change problems.

MI works by activating patients' own motivation for change and adherence to treatment. Patients exposed to MI (vs. treatment as usual) have been found in various clinical trials to be more likely to enter, stay in, and complete treatment; to participate in follow-up visits; to adhere to glucose monitoring and to improve glycemic control; to increase exercise and fruit and vegetable intake; to reduce stress and sodium intake; to keep food diaries; to reduce unprotected sex and needle sharing; to improve medication adherence; to decrease alcohol and illicit drug use; to quit smoking; and to have fewer subsequent injuries and hospitalizations. It is not a panacea, of course; not all trials have been positive, and the size of effect has varied widely. Readers interested in the research base can find a bibliography of outcome studies at the back of this book and also at *www.motivationalinterview.org*.

MI works by activating patients' own motivation for change and adherence to treatment.

THE MYTH OF THE UNMOTIVATED PATIENT

Conversations about behavior change arise within a consultation whenever you or your patients are considering their *doing* something different in the interest of health. That "doing" might be taking a medication regularly, using a walker, flossing teeth, changing diet, exercising, and so on. It might also involve cutting down or quitting behaviors that are harmful to health: smoking, heavy drinking, drug abuse, overworking, or eating junk food. Across health care specialties, the scope of possible health behavior change that can be discussed broadens considerably to include such subjects as patients' footwear (in diabetes), fluid intake (kidney disease), condom use, attendance at a clinic, use of hearing aids, and so on. For the purposes of this book, a strict definition of health behavior might not be necessary.

Conversations about behavior change arise whenever you or your patients are considering their doing something different in the interest of health.

When a patient seems unmotivated to change or to take the sound

When a patient seems unmotivated to change or to take the sound advice of practitioners, it is often assumed that there is something the matter with the patient and that there is not much one can do about it. These assumptions are usually false. No person is completely unmotivated.

advice of practitioners, it is often assumed that there is something the matter with the patient and that there is not much one can do about it. These assumptions are usually false. A starting point for this book is that motivation for change is actually quite malleable and is particularly formed in the context of relationships.

The way in which you talk with patients about their health can substantially influence their personal motivation for behavior change. No person is completely unmotivated. We all have goals and aspirations. You can make a difference and have a long-term influence on your patients' health. How, then, should one respond when what patients need is behavior and lifestyle change?

The way in which you talk with patients about their health can substantially influence their personal motivation for behavior change.

THE "SPIRIT" OF MI

MI is not a technique for tricking people into doing what they do not want to do. Rather, it is a skillful clinical style for eliciting from patients their own good motivations for making behavior changes in the interest of their health. It involves guiding more than directing, dancing rather than wrestling, listening at least as much as telling. The overall "spirit" has been described as *collaborative*, *evocative*, and *honoring of patient autonomy*.

- *Collaborative*. MI rests on a cooperative and collaborative partnership between patient and clinician. Whereas the patient-centered clinical method is a broad approach to the consultation, MI addresses the specific situation in which patient behavior change is needed. Instead of an uneven power relationship in which the expert clinician directs the passive patient in what to do, there is an active collaborative conversation and joint decision-making process. This is particularly vital in health behavior change, because ultimately it is only the patient who can enact such change.
- *Evocative*. Often health care seems to involve giving patients what they lack, be it medication, knowledge, insight, or skills. MI instead seeks to evoke from patients that which they already have, to activate their own motivation and resources for change. A patient may not be motivated to do what you want him or her to, but each person has personal goals, values, aspirations, and dreams. Part of the art of MI is connecting health behavior change with what your patients care about, with their own values and concerns. This can be done only by under-

standing patients' own perspectives, by evoking their own good reasons and arguments for change.

Often health care seems to involve giving patients what they lack, be it medication, knowledge, insight, or skills. MI instead seeks to evoke from patients that which they already have.

- *Honoring patient autonomy.* MI also requires a certain degree of detachment from outcomes—not an absence of caring, but rather an acceptance that people can and do make choices about the course of their lives. Clinicians may inform, advise, even warn, but ultimately it is the patient who decides what to do. To recognize and honor this autonomy is also a key element in facilitating health behavior change. There is something in human nature that resists being coerced and told what to do. Ironically, it is acknowledging the other's right and freedom not to change that sometimes makes change possible.

There is something in human nature that resists being coerced and told what to do. Ironically, it is acknowledging the other's right and freedom not to change that sometimes makes change possible.

These three characteristics describe the underlying "spirit" of MI, the mindset with which one approaches conversations with patients about behavior change.

FOUR GUIDING PRINCIPLES

Relatedly, the practice of MI has four guiding principles: (1) to resist the righting reflex, (2) to understand and explore the patient's own motivations, (3) to listen with empathy, and (4) to empower the patient, encouraging hope and optimism. These four principles can be remembered by the acronym RULE: Resist, Understand, Listen, and Empower.

R: Resist the Righting Reflex

People who enter helping professions often have a powerful desire to set things right, to heal, to prevent harm and promote well-being. When seeing someone headed down the wrong path, they will usually want to get out in front of the person and say, "Stop! Turn back! There is a better way!" This is a laudable motivation; it is often what calls people into service to others. Given this motivation, the urge to correct another's course often becomes automatic, almost reflexive.

A problem is that this first inclination can have a paradoxical effect. The reason is not that patients are flawed, recalcitrant, lazy, or in the grip of pernicious denial. Rather, it is a natural human tendency to resist persuasion. This is particularly true when one is ambivalent about something. Problem drinkers, for example, often know perfectly well that they are drinking too much and that it is having some adverse consequences. But they also enjoy drinking and don't like to think of themselves as "having a problem," and thus they prefer to see their drinking as reasonably normal. Virtually every problem drinker we have treated, if allowed to explore it, has felt two ways about drinking.

When a health professional takes up the "good" side of the patient's internal argument and tries to set the patient right, what happens? If you say, "I think you are drinking too much, and should cut down or quit," the patient's natural response is to argue the other side of the ambivalence: "It's not that bad, and I'm doing fine." The temptation then is to turn up the volume, to argue all the more forcefully that the person is in trouble and needs to make a change. The patient's response, again, is predictable.

PRACTITIONER: Well, if you did decide to exercise more, that would not only help your knee but also help you lose weight and improve your mood, you know. Exercise makes people slimmer, fitter, and feel better.

PATIENT: Yes, I know all that. But I can't help thinking that if I exercise while my knee hurts, even with gentle things like swimming, that I am doing more damage to it, despite what you say about those studies you read. . . .

This acting out of the patient's internal dilemma might be therapeutic in some way were it not for another well-documented basic principle of human nature: We tend to believe what we hear ourselves say. The more patients verbalize the disadvantages of change, the more committed they become to sustaining the status quo. If you converse in a way that causes patients to defend the status quo and argue against change, you may well inadvertently decrease rather than increase the likelihood of behavior change actually happening.

We tend to believe what we hear ourselves say. The more patients verbalize the disadvantages of change, the more committed they become to sustaining the status quo.

In sum, if you are arguing for change and your patient is resisting and arguing against it, you're in the wrong role. You are taking all the good lines. It is the *patient* who should be voicing the arguments for change. MI is about evoking those arguments from the patient, and that means first suppressing what may seem like the right thing to do—the righting reflex.

On many, if not most, issues of health behavior change, patients are ambivalent. They want to; they might be able to; they see good reasons to; they know they need to; and then they hit that "but." That's where patients' thinking may stop unless you help them through the ambivalence. Fortunately, there is much you can do to make that happen, starting with the next guiding principle.

U: Understand Your Patient's Motivations

It is the patient's own reasons for change, and not yours, that are most likely to trigger behavior change. And so a second guiding principle is to be interested in the patient's own concerns, values, and motivations. In MI one proceeds in a way that evokes and explores patients' perceptions about their current situations and their own motivations for change. This may sound like a prolonged process, but it need not be. It can be done within the normal length of your consultation. We believe, in fact, that if your consultation time is limited, you are better off asking patients why they would want to make a change and how they might do it rather than telling them that they should. It is the patient, rather than you, who should be voicing the arguments for behavior change. We address the practicalities, the "how to," of this and other principles in Part II.

If your consultation time is limited, you are better off asking patients why they would want to make a change and how they might do it rather than telling them that they should.

L: Listen to Your Patient

MI involves at least as much listening as informing. Perhaps the normal expectations of a health care consultation are that the practitioner has the answers and will give them to the patients. Often you do have answers, and patients come to you for this expertise. When it comes to behavior change, though, the answers most likely lie within the patient, and finding them requires some listening.

Good listening is actually a complex clinical skill. It requires more than asking questions and keeping quiet long though to hear patients' replies. In their book *Making the Patient Your Partner*, psychologist Thomas Gordon and surgeon Sterling Edwards discussed how such quality listening is a vital part of good medical care in general.* It involves an empathic interest in making sure you understand, making guesses about meaning—a skill discussed in more detail in Chapter 5.

---

* Gordon, T., & Edwards, W. S. (1995). *Making the patient your partner: Communication skills for doctors and other caregivers*. Westport, CT: Auburn House.

E: Empower Your Patient

It is increasingly clear that outcomes are better when patients take an active interest and role in their own health care. A fourth guiding principle in MI is empowerment—helping patients explore how they *can* make a difference in their own health. Again, the patient's own ideas and resources are key here. You know that regular exercise is important, but it is your patients who know best how they could successfully build it into their daily lives. Patients in essence become your consultants on their own lives and on how best to accomplish behavior change. An important role for you in this process is to support their hope that such change is possible and can make a difference in their health. A patient who is active in the consultation, thinking aloud about the why and how of change, is more likely to do something about this afterward. You, the practitioner, are an expert in facilitating the patients' bringing their expertise to the consultation.

A patient who is active in the consultation, thinking aloud about the why and how of change, is more likely to do something about this afterward.

Encouraging health behavior change by applying MI effectively within the space of a few minutes and in conjunction with other health care tasks is a highly skillful process. Through working in health care and listening to countless consultations over the years, we have developed deep admiration for the level of skillfulness that so many frontline clinicians already manifest in practice each and every day. Our hope in providing this book is not to displace these naturally honed skills and instincts but rather to offer what assistance we can in supporting your desire and ability to help patients change.

CONCLUSION

This chapter has described the rationale for using MI when talking to patients about behavior change. In the next chapters we discuss in more detail how MI fits into the normal communication processes of health care. Chapter 2 places the *guiding* style within a continuum of communication styles that you normally use in practice. We describe MI as a refined form of guiding. We also discuss three core communication skills that are also part of normal practice. The purpose of all of this is to help you place MI within the context of your day-to-day work. In Part II we explain how these basic skills can be used in the service of guiding behavior change.

CHAPTER 2

How Motivational Interviewing Fits into Health Care Practice

How do you take MI, developed by psychologists for counseling, and use it in your everyday practice? Your time is often short, and we are asking you to absorb not just technical matters but also a different way of thinking about promoting change in others. MI can seem both comfortingly familiar and difficult to integrate. Is it something completely different from what you do normally? Our answer is no.

This chapter aims to link MI and everyday health care practice through examination of three common styles of communication in health care: directing, guiding, and following. MI is a refined form of guiding. In this chapter we also look at three core communication skills: asking, informing, and listening. These skills are simple and basic in themselves, but, used in combination, they are the tools that make for either effective or ineffective directing, guiding, and following.

MI can seem both comfortingly familiar and difficult to integrate. Is it something completely different from what you do normally? Our answer is no.

"BUT I USE THIS METHOD EVERY DAY . . . "

"This MI method is nothing new. I do this every day." This is a common reaction among practitioners who are presented with a description of MI for the first time. You may have recognized explanations and even recalled recent consultations characterized by some of the principles described in Chapter 1. Perhaps a patient was talking about behavior change in a constructive way, and your role seemed almost effortless. Perhaps you were not trying to convince the patient to change at all. Your role was a quieter, more supportive one. As the 17th-century French polymath Blaise Pascal wrote in his *Pensées*, "People are generally better persuaded by the reasons which they have themselves discovered than by those which have come in to the mind of others." Indeed, eliciting motivation for change from patients themselves is not a new idea, and neither is the supportive approach that we call guiding. MI is built on this platform.

THREE COMMUNICATION STYLES

One of the most striking features of MI is a feeling that you get in the consultation, almost tangible, that your stance in relation to the patient is easy and less conflict-ridden. As a colleague once remarked, "It's like dancing rather than wrestling." This experience is not just a reflection of the patient's attitude and behavior but of yours as well. It is linked to how you approach the whole topic of behavior change. Shift your style, and the consultation feels different.

The term "style" captures nicely this strategic approach to helping patients. In this book a communication style refers to an attitude and approach to helping patients, a way of talking with them that characterizes your relationship with them. Different communication styles are used for different purposes. The guiding style seems particularly suited to difficult conversations about behavior change. However, other styles are better suited to other purposes. Here are some concrete examples.

Imagine that you are sitting down with a good friend to talk over something that is distressing her. In particular, she is torn about whether to stay in a relationship with someone she has cared about for years. It's a decision with far-reaching implications. How will you respond?

One approach is to listen carefully and follow along as she pours out her story, seeking to be sympathetic and supportive as she sorts out what she wants to do. By listening and taking the time to understand what she is experiencing, you are also helping her to voice and clarify her own feelings. You don't offer any answers for her. Rather, you try to be a good companion on this journey that is clearly hers to make.

Suppose, however, that you have a very clear opinion as to what she should do. A second approach would be to offer your straightforward advice as her close friend. By telling her how you see her situation, making a clear suggestion, and explaining your rationale for it, you hope to be helpful in getting her unstuck and moving in a healthier and happier direction. In this approach you respond to a person in distress by telling her what she should (or at least could) do, helping her solve her problem.

A third approach goes down the middle between the other two, combining some of the better qualities of both. You listen carefully and empathically to understand your friend's dilemma. Then you ask her about the various options she is considering, and you both explore together the pros and cons of each. Here or there you may offer a bit of what you know about her or about people and relationships more generally, recognizing and honoring that ultimately it is her life and her decision to make. As some clarity emerges, you help her to move in the direction that she has chosen.

These three examples correspond, respectively, to the three communication styles to be discussed in this chapter: following, directing, and guiding. All three are legitimate and important methods of communication. All three are used in everyday life, as well as in health care practice, and each style has contexts in which it fits and works best. We therefore make no value judgments about the worthiness of each style. Instead, we suggest that problems emerge when there is an incongruity between style and task. One way of thinking about these three styles is to imagine them along a continuum, with following at one end, directing at the other, and guiding in the middle. Another is to imagine that you are sitting in the center of a circle, able to reach out to use the appropriate style as needed (see Figure 2.1).

In a way, each of these styles reflects different attitudes about your role in the relationship. For a helping professional, they reflect different

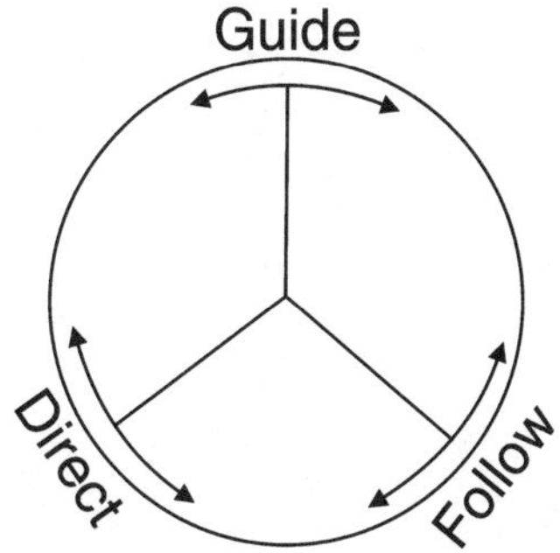

FIGURE 2.1. Three communication styles.

assumptions about how one is to go about the process of being helpful in different situations.

Following

Everyone likes a good listener, and most people believe that they are good listeners. A truly good listener suspends his or her own "stuff" in the interest of giving full attention to understanding the other's experience. Good listening does not involve instructing or directing, agreeing or disagreeing, persuading or advising, warning or analyzing. It has no agenda to achieve other than seeing and understanding the world through the other's eyes.

In the style of following, listening predominates. You follow the other person's lead. With regard to behavior change, a following style communicates "I won't change or push you. I trust your wisdom about yourself, and I'll let you work this out in your own time and at your own pace." A patient who is in tears after you deliver bad news needs a following style from you. So, too, at the beginning of a consultation, a brief period of following helps you to understand patients' symptoms and how these fit into the larger picture of their life and health.

Some synonyms for "following":	
Go along with	*Go after*
Allow	*Attend*
Permit	*Take in*
Be responsive	*Shadow*
Have faith in	*Understand*
	Observe

Directing

The directing style bespeaks quite a different interpersonal relationship. In this approach you take charge, at least for the time being. It implies an uneven relationship with regard to knowledge, expertise, authority, or power. Sometimes this approach saves lives. A director, in essence, tells a person what to do, with or without explaining the rationale. In everyday life, a director is usually responsible for seeing that you perform your job properly, for judging your performance, and for overseeing appropriate consequences for a job well or poorly done. There are, of course, other styles of management, but a clear line of authority is involved in being a director, man-

Some synonyms for "directing":	
Manage	*Prescribe*
Lead	*Tell*
Take charge	*Show the way*
Preside	*Govern*
Rule	*Authorize*
Reign	*Take the reins*
Conduct	*Take command*
Determine	*Point toward*
Steer	*Administer*

ager, supervisor, or chief. With regard to behavior change, the directing style communicates, "I know how you can solve this problem. I know what you should do." The expected complementary role is adherence or compliance. Many health care practitioners will recognize this as one of the cornerstones of their education. A directing style seems appropriate for countless situations in which a patient depends on you for decisions, action, and advice. Patients often appear to expect and want this kind of take-charge approach from you.

Guiding

A guide helps you find your way. It is not within the guide's authority to determine what you want to see or do. You decide where to go, and you hire a knowledgeable guide or travel agent to help you get there. Consider the guide and director roles in education. In a director role, medical faculty determine what their students will study, what learning activities are required, and what standards constitute acceptable performance. A more guiding role is that of a tutor, who is a resource to help students in more self-directed learning. A good guide knows what is possible and can offer you alternatives from which to choose. With regard to behavior change, the guiding style communicates, "I can help you to solve this for yourself."

Some synonyms for "guiding":

Enlighten	*Look after*
Encourage	*Take along*
Motivate	*Accompany*
Support	*Awaken*
Lay before	*Elicit*

With regard to behavior change, the guiding style communicates, "I can help you to solve this for yourself."

Mix and Match

All three of these styles—following, directing, and guiding—are used in everyday life. They are suited to different types of circumstances and relationships, and a mismatch can cause problems. A student who takes a directing tone with a teacher is stepping out of role and may thereby get into trouble. A parent who follows along passively while a wild child rampages around a restaurant is likely to be regarded as irresponsible.

More often these three communication styles are intermixed, and skillfulness in communication in-

All three of these styles—following, directing, and guiding—are used in everyday life. They are suited to different types of circumstances and relationships, and a mismatch can cause problems.

volves flexible shifting among them. Watch a skillful parent and young child for an hour, and you will probably see all three styles. Good parenting requires good following—being willing and able to listen to a child's feelings and imagination, hopes and fears, successes and adventures. Good parenting also requires some directing, such as when a child is about to wander out into traffic on a busy street. The setting of consistent limits involves directing: "Get out of the bath now!" "Homework first, then we'll play."

Skillful parents also guide. By the age of 6 or so, children ordinarily develop the ability to self-regulate, to form a plan and direct their behavior toward it without external enforcement. Children vary widely, however, in the extent to which they can self-regulate, and parenting style is a contributing factor. Research shows that parents whose children develop solid self-regulation skills tend to use a guiding style in helping their children to learn. Imagine a parent and a 4-year-old child seated together at a table. The child's task is to use the various-sized blocks on the table to build a tower as tall as possible. What does the parent do? The *directing* parent tells the child what to do at every step along the way, immediately corrects mistakes, and may even take over block placement for the child: "Let me do that!" The *following* parent sits back and watches the child's trial and error without offering help. The *guiding* parent does a little of both: watching patiently and with interest, but also stepping in now and then perhaps to whisper a tip in the child's ear—"Try putting the big ones on the bottom!"—then stepping back again to let the child try.

An art teacher could similarly work anywhere along this continuum. A highly directing teacher might ask the student to copy step by step or might literally hold and direct the hand that holds the brush or chisel. A following teacher might provide the raw materials and then sit back, letting students explore freely without direction. In between is the guiding style, in which the art teacher walks around the room, watching attentively, providing encouragement, asking what the student has in mind, now and then offering a suggestion if the student wants it. The same teacher may use all three styles flexibly within the same class session or may begin with more directing early in the course and then step back to more guiding and following as students progress.

Think back to your own favorite teacher—the one in whose class you were particularly motivated and engaged, the one who saw possibilities and brought out the best in you. Though it is not always the case, this person was probably skillful at guiding you.

Across the wide range of circumstances you meet in everyday health care practice, there is a place for each style. A skillful practitioner is someone able to shift flexibly among these styles as appropriate to the patient and situation. What is described as "an old-fashioned, good bedside manner" is probably a reflection of much more than a friendly doctor or nurse. It is someone with the skill to switch among communication styles and the wisdom to seek and understand what style the patient needs.

A skillful practitioner is someone able to shift flexibly among these styles as appropriate to the patient and situation.

The Overuse of Directing

Skillful practitioners abound, and they often seem like the unsung heroes in the maelstrom of modern clinical practice. Yet a disturbing pattern seems evident in health care, in both practice and management, with the balance of communication shifting toward directing while the value of following and guiding is often ignored. The well-intentioned efforts of service providers to assess, prioritize, diagnose, provide, measure, promote, follow up, and reach targets can express themselves in a directing style that compromises quality care, permeates most conversations, and all too often renders patients the passive recipients of doses of care. Under pressures of time to check off boxes, conduct standardized assessments, adhere to competency frameworks, and reduce costs, an action-oriented culture sometimes prevails, and directing is the style that expresses this value. The difficulty, however, is that many problems are more effectively solved by a better balanced mixture of styles. It is often better to follow and contemplate a little, to support and guide, before using a directing style.

A disturbing pattern seems evident in health care, with the balance of communication shifting toward directing rather than following and guiding.

> Stefan is 14-year-old boy who attends the diabetes clinic every few months, where he goes through a routine of weight and blood glucose testing with familiar, friendly faces. He has failed to bring his diary along (was he even keeping it properly?). His meeting with the doctor starts with some friendly chat, then proceeds through a series of investigative questions to the main concern: a poor blood glucose test result. He is strongly advised to keep his diary more faithfully and to maintain a good injecting routine. He leaves feeling guilty. He did not expect his struggles with puberty and diabetes to be raised, and they weren't. But at least on this occasion, he wasn't told to watch his diet and get more regular exercise. That was a relief.

A directing style is appropriate in many circumstances and can be used skillfully, but it ought not to be the only way you interact with patients. There are times when it is not essential or even possible for you to be the expert director, and that is particularly true in discussions of patients' lifestyle and behavior change, in which it is crucial to engage the patient's own motivation, energy, and commitment. A guiding style is probably called for, something Stefan might have responded to better. If you want cooperative patients, directing is not your only option.

There are times when it is not essential or even possible for you to be the expert director, and that is particularly true in discussions of patients' lifestyle and behavior change, in which it is crucial to engage the patient's own motivation, energy, and commitment. A guiding style is probably called for.

Guiding, MI, and Behavior Change

Health care ethics emphasize human autonomy, the right of the person to make informed decisions about the course of his or her own life. Much as one might like to step in and make the "right" choices for a patient (or child, or student), the practitioner's ability to do so is constrained. Health outcomes are often highly influenced by and dependent on the patient's own behavioral choices—on doing something new or differently. Smoking, drinking, diet, exercise, medication adherence—these are examples of important health behaviors that can have a major effect on the course of a patient's health or illness and over which health care practitioners have little or no direct control. Yet letting go of some control does not mean lack of influence. In human relationships, it is quite possible to influence that which we do not personally control.

Guiding is well suited to helping people solve behavior-change problems. MI is a refined form of this guiding style. A practitioner using MI will conduct the discussion in line with a guiding style, *paying particular attention to how to help the patient make his or her own decisions about behavior change.* Thus, although all MI could be considered a form of guiding, not all guiding is MI! In contrast to the more general guiding style, MI:

Guiding is well suited to helping people solve behavior-change problems. MI is a refined form of this guiding style.

- Is specifically goal-directed. Often the practitioner has a specific behavior-change goal in mind and gently guides the pa-

tient to consider why and how he or she might pursue that goal.
- Pays particular attention to certain aspects of patient language and actively seeks to evoke the patient's own arguments for change.
- Involves competence in a well-defined set of clinical skills and strategies that are used to evoke patient behavior change.

To help you understand the heart and nature of this way of talking with patients, we next look at three basic communication skills. Used in combination, these skills are your tools for creating the communication styles we have been discussing, including MI.

THREE CORE COMMUNICATION SKILLS

Asking, informing, and listening are three basic but important communication skills. They are the means by which any of the three communication styles just discussed can be put into practice. These skills are observable behaviors, the things that you actually do to implement the style you are adopting. Health professionals regularly ask, listen to, and inform patients in their consultations. Using these tools well increases your freedom to conduct the consultation in a time-efficient and productive manner. They are the communication equivalent of technical proficiency in music; the more proficient, the wider the range of application, skillfulness, and enjoyment. Here is a brief synopsis of each skill:

- *Asking*. The practitioner's intent in asking questions is usually to develop an understanding of the patient's problem(s). Some nuances, functions, and consequences of using this tool within a guiding style are described in Chapter 4.
- *Listening*. Good listening is an active process. It is a check on whether you understand the person's meaning correctly, and it also communicates "What you are saying is important to me. I want to hear more." Done well, it also encourages the patient to explore and reveal more, and it sometimes does so within a surprisingly short period of time. In many ways, good listening is the core skill when using the guiding style.

Asking, listening, and informing are the communication equivalent of technical proficiency in music; the more proficient, the wider the range of application, skillfulness, and enjoyment.

- *Informing*. The principal vehicle for conveying knowledge to the patient about a condition and its treatment is informing. The practitioner usually informs the patient about a range of facts, diagnoses, and recommendations. When informing is not done well it can result in poor adherence or glazed looks from patients as the practitioner talks to them.

What Is Your Preference?

Of these three core communication skills, is there one that you particularly favor in practice? You do use all three, of course, but perhaps you tend to rely on one of these more than others in talking with your patients. Practitioners tend to develop consistent habits in health care consultations. Do your consultations tend to lean more heavily on one of these communication tools, or perhaps a combination of two out of the three? The same question applies to the three communication styles described earlier. Do your current consultations lean more toward directing, guiding, or following?

Practitioners tend to develop consistent habits in health care consultations. Do your consultations tend to lean more heavily on one of these communication tools, or perhaps a combination of two out of the three?

When we ask which tools practitioners use most, the most common answer we hear is, "Asking and then informing," and practitioners report using these skills mostly in the service of a directing style. For example, "I find out what's wrong with the patient [asking and listening], then I diagnose and recommend treatment [informing]." This one–two–three combination is obviously useful in practice, but when it comes to behavior change, it also contains some unintended consequences; more on this later.

One practitioner we met reacted with consternation to the possibility of incorporating some new evidence about the management of a particular problem. "Oh, no," he laughed. "Now I'm going to have to develop a completely new line of patter." Then he explained that he had developed a very comfortable routine for managing his consultations. He asked a few questions about specific symptoms and then delivered information, suited to the circumstances, about diagnosis and treatment. This was his *modus operandi*. It involved mostly asking and informing, and he could do it in his sleep. Now he felt obliged to consider broadening his repertoire. His "line of patter," as well as his attitude toward helping his patients, began to change.

STYLES AND SKILLS: YOUR ATTITUDE AND YOUR BEHAVIOR

All three skills (asking, listening, informing) are used in all three styles (following, guiding, directing), but the skill mix in each style may be quite different. The key difference among the three styles is in the underlying attitude and assumptions about how to address a patient's problem. Of course, your attitude is not expressed just in the skill mix but also by complementary signals from your tone of voice, the quality of eye contact, body language, and such things as the seating arrangement in your consulting room.

Figure 2.2 presents a model of the relationship between styles and skills. In general, the directing style tends to be heavy on informing, whereas a following style relies heavily on listening. All three styles involve a certain amount of asking. The guiding style features perhaps the most equitable balance in use of the three tools.

Asking in the service of directing will often look and sound quite different from asking in the service of a following or a guiding style. Similarly with listening and informing.

Figure 2.2 describes the *frequency* with which skills might be used across styles. However, there is another important difference across styles: the way in which they are used and the purposes they are used for. Thus asking in the service of directing will often look and sound quite different from asking in the service of a following or a guiding

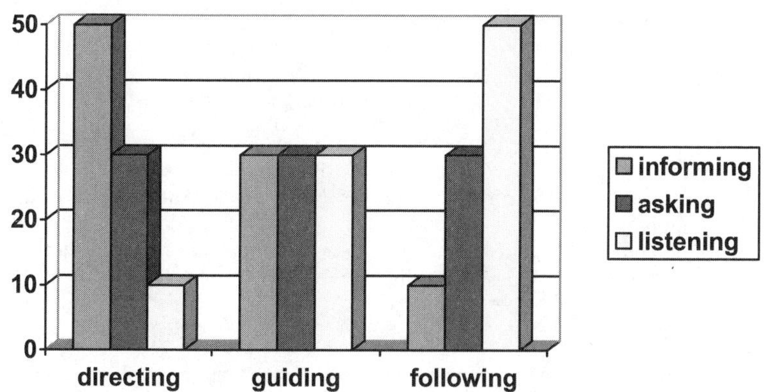

FIGURE 2.2. Styles and skills: How often are skills used within different styles? Adapted with permission from Barbara B. Walker.

style. So, too, with listening and informing. As an example of the skill of asking, "How much do you smoke each day?" is often phrased in a way that's indicative of a directing style, whereas "What would it take for you to stop smoking?" might be more indicative of a guiding style. Table 2.1 provides more examples.

Directing and Core Skills

A directing style can be just what patients expect and well suited to the demands of the clinical situation. Done well, directing has a quality of being well timed, personally relevant, clear, and compassionate. To achieve this, you might have to begin with a following style.

Done well, directing has a quality of being well timed, personally relevant, clear and compassionate. . . . It can also be used with a lack of grace.

Poor Directing

Directing can also be used with a lack of grace, in a way that leaves patients feeling unheard and dissatisfied. Here is an example of directing gone wrong. A patient with a hip problem consults a specialist who has the latest X-ray results:

TABLE 2.1. Asking, Informing, and Listening Vary According to the Style Being Used

Asking

- "How may times has that happened?" [directing]
- "What kind of change makes sense to you?" [guiding]
- "How have you been since your son died?" [following]

Informing

- "Your best option is to take these tablets." [directing]
- "Changing your diet would make sense medically, but how does that feel for you?" [guiding]
- "Yes, it's a common experience; many patients also feel quite shocked and unsettled about simple things like going to the toilet." [following]

Listening

- "So you understand what's going to happen this morning, but you want me to tell you more about what will happen later on." [directing]
- "You're feeling concerned about your weight, and you are not sure where to go from here." [guiding]
- "This has been a huge shock." [following]

PRACTITIONER: How have you been getting along with the hip? [asking]

PATIENT: Well, since that operation its been really hellish, to be honest. The pain is still really hard to bear and sometimes those pills just don't help. I wonder if there is something still wrong with it.

PRACTITIONER: Have you been in to see your family doctor? [asking]

PATIENT: Yes, she's given me these pills that she said you recommended.

PRACTITIONER: Good, because I think they will help you. I can tell you that the X-ray shows that you have made a very good recovery and that your hip appears to be in good condition. [informing]

PATIENT: Well, uh, it still hurts so much, I tell you, doctor, yesterday it was unbearable.

PRACTITIONER: It will get better with time, if you are doing all the right things like I told you. Take your medication and take a walk twice a day. I'd like to see you again in 3 months. [informing]

PATIENT: Yes, OK, but have you any idea why it hurts so much?

PRACTITIONER: Well, my examination of your hip and the X-ray tells me that the hip is healing, and sometimes this just takes time. [informing]

PATIENT: Is there any other medicine that might help?

PRACTITIONER: Well, we've got you on the best medicine we can give you. The process of mobilization is often painful to begin with. We could arrange some extra physical therapy for you if you like. I'll sort it out. You'll get a letter or a telephone call within the next week or so.

In this example, the practitioner exclusively used a directing style, with a lack of listening. This suggested a lack of interest in the patient as a person and even communicated disrespect. It also undermined the opportunity to gain important diagnostic information.

Better Directing

The habitual use of an "ask–inform, ask–inform" pattern of skill usage can be quite off-putting to patients. It can be done differently (the same scenario as preceding):

PRACTITIONER: How have you been getting along with the hip? [asking]

PATIENT: Well, since that operation its been really hellish, to be honest.

The pain is still really hard to bear and sometimes those pills just don't help. I wonder if there is something still wrong with it?

PRACTITIONER: It sounds like you are going through a difficult time. [listening]

PATIENT: Terrible. I mean I expected pain, but there's something about this that doesn't feel right, so much so that my son is convinced that something went wrong in the operation, and he says I must ask you about this.

PRACTITIONER: I honestly don't think so, when I look at your hip itself and the X-ray [informing], but tell me, when and how does it hurt? [asking]

PATIENT: You see, I have taken the tablets that you and my family doctor recommended, but it's no good. When I get up from my chair or bed, it's really terrible. I don't complain easily.

PRACTITIONER: Let's have a look at the X-ray together. If you look just here, what we look for is whether the new joint is in the right place and the bones are all OK, and on this one of yours it looks fine.

PATIENT: So you don't see a problem there?

PRACTITIONER: No. Mobilization after these operations can sometimes be pretty tough, but if you soldier on, I think it will get better [informing]. But it sounds like you will feel more reassured if we keep a much more careful eye on your progress and arrange for some extra help with getting you properly going again.

PATIENT: I'd really appreciate that.

PRACTITIONER: I will ask for the physical therapist to see you again to help you more with that. She will be able to guide you about that tough trade-off between pain and activity. [informing]

PATIENT: So you don't think there is anything really wrong with my hip?

PRACTITIONER: Based on what I see here, it doesn't seem like it, but I do think we need to keep a close eye on your progress. [informing]

PATIENT: Is there any other medicine that might help?

(*The patient and practitioner discuss medicine and physical therapy assessment and support.*)

The small increase in listening, based on a genuine desire to take on board the concerns and experiences of the patient, clearly enriches the

The small increase in listening, based on a genuine desire to take on board the concerns and experiences of the patient, clearly enriches the use of a directing style and the diagnostic task.

diagnostic task. The use of a directing style in this example leaves the patient feeling better understood and, indeed, with a more helpful plan for his or her recovery.

Following and Core Skills

Following and Gathering Information

It is easy to appreciate the value of a following style when working with a patient facing distressing circumstances. However, probably more common is the use of this style at the beginning of the consultation:

PRACTITIONER: How are things going?

PATIENT: Well, not so good, to be honest, I've been in a lot of pain.

PRACTITIONER: Tell me what's happened. [asking]

PATIENT: Well it's one thing to have arthritis, another thing to be having this. (*Bends to one side, rubs left knee.*)

PRACTITIONER: I can see that you're in pain now, as you speak. [listening]

PATIENT: Yes, I am, and it's driving me crazy, slowly but surely.

PRACTITIONER: It's one thing to have the arthritis you've had for some time, but this is something different. [listening]

PATIENT: No, it's not different, it's the same damn knee, but the pain is now too much.

PRACTITIONER: It's getting hard for you to bear, and it's dominating your life. [listening]

PATIENT: Exactly. My wife drove me down here, but you should see how I hobbled into the clinic.

PRACTITIONER: Tell me about what this pain is like and how it's affecting you. [asking]

PATIENT: Well, I don't know. I can hardly get out of the chair. I can't go down to the shops any more. Even if I got there, the pain is just eating me up . . .

PRACTITIONER: Most of the time, this pain is there and it's gnawing away at you. [listening]

PATIENT: That's a good word, because it's always there, slowly driving me crazy.

(*The discussion continues, and the patient talks about how it's affecting almost every part of his life.*)

PRACTITIONER: (*shifting style to directing*) Can I ask you now about pain relief? Tell me, . . . [asking]

Following a Request for Treatment

Following is also an appropriate style when a patient makes a request and it is appropriate for you to go along with this.

PATIENT: I've heard about those patches to help you quit smoking. I want to give them a try. Will you prescribe them for me?

PRACTITIONER: You really want to quit. [listening]

PATIENT: I do. I've made the decision, and tomorrow is the day, if you can let me have those patches.

PRACTITIONER: Good for you. You feel that patches is the right way to go. [listening]

PATIENT: Yes, I cannot go cold turkey without nicotine replacement. I tried that before. I felt sick, even vomited once, jumpy, I just couldn't cope. Another time, I even tried hypnosis. What a waste of money that was. My partner tried the patches and they worked for him. I think I want to try them, too.

PRACTITIONER: So it's worked for your partner and you are determined to do so as well. [listening]

PATIENT: Yeah. If he can do it, so can I. In some ways he was more addicted than me. He's really supportive now, and together I think we can beat it this time.

PRACTITIONER: Great. I just need to check a few things with you . . . [informing]

Following an Upset Patient

Most practitioners would agree that following is highly recommended when a patient is distressed, angry, or very anxious.

PATIENT: I'm shattered. I think you know that they told me yesterday that I will probably die in just a matter of months.

PRACTITIONER: This must have come to you as quite a shock. [listening]

PATIENT: A terrible shock. I was afraid of this (*bursts into tears*).

PRACTITIONER: Your worst fears were confirmed. [listening]

PATIENT: Exactly. It's not like I hadn't thought of this before, but to hear someone actually say it, just like that. I was stunned.

PRACTITIONER: You wish the news had been broken to you more gently. [listening]

PATIENT: No, I knew, really, as soon as I saw his face. I just keep hearing him say it over and over again.

PRACTITIONER: You're lying here, alone most of the time, with this running through your mind. [listening]

PATIENT: It's terrible. I just don't know what to do.

PRACTITIONER: Is there anything I can do to help? [asking]

PATIENT: No, I don't think so. It's just such a shock. Thank you for asking.

PRACTITIONER: Well, I'll be here most of the day today, and I'll pop in and see you a little later. I know that your pain medication needs reviewing, and I'd like to talk to you about this. [informing]

Guiding and Core Skills

Next we present a brief example of how the three core skills can be used in the service of guiding. Parts II and III of this book contain many more examples of guiding.

Encouraging a Referral

Helping a patient with a referral to another colleague is an example of behavior change. The motivation to actually attend a new appointment can be influenced by your communication style. In this case, the practitioner (a social worker, nurse, counselor, doctor) would like to refer a patient with diabetes to a dietician for consultation about cooking and eating habits. One approach might be to simply tell the patient, "You need to go see the dietician for advice about your eating habits. Here is the number to call." How might this same task be approached within a guiding style?

PRACTITIONER: From your lab tests, your blood sugar level is still high, and that worries me. [informing] If you're willing to take a few minutes to talk about this, could you tell me a little about your eating habits? [asking]

PATIENT: Well, I try to be careful, and I stay away from sweets and junk food mostly.

PRACTITIONER: You're avoiding some foods that really drive up your blood sugar. [listening] What about fixing food at home? [asking]

PATIENT: I do most of the cooking for the family. Everybody likes different things, so it's a challenge. I could probably do a little better there in preparing healthier meals.

PRACTITIONER: You see a little possible room for improvement in how you cook. [listening]

PATIENT: Yes, I think so.

PRACTITIONER: That's a common challenge for people with diabetes, and a good place to think about making some changes. Would you like a little help with thinking about ways to fix food that would help you manage your diabetes? [asking]

PATIENT: I think I know the basics, but sure, I could learn more.

PRACTITIONER: Good! I can tell you a little here, but we have staff who really specialize in helping people with diabetes think about how they cook and eat. [informing] How would you feel about talking with somebody knowledgeable like that? [asking]

PATIENT: I guess so. I work during the day, though, and I had to take off time to come see you today.

PRACTITIONER: You're willing to give it a try, particularly if you could come in at a time that doesn't interfere with work. [listening]

PATIENT: Yes. I mean, I couldn't get here often during the day, but after work would help.

PRACTITIONER: OK, good. I know they have some evening times available. [informing] Let's call over there and see when they can fit you in. Would that be OK? [asking]

PATIENT: Sure.

Taking an extra minute to negotiate a referral in a guiding style may make all the difference in whether the patient actually gets there. Placing the call yourself or asking a colleague to do it while the patient is still in the building also significantly enhances a referral. This short exchange illustrated three of the principles of motivational interviewing noted in Chapter 1: understanding the patient's motivation, listening, and empowering the patient. The outcome, reflected in the patient's responses, was change talk, a topic discussed in detail in the next chapter. Attendance at the referral is more likely to take place.

FLEXIBILITY WITHIN A CONSULTATION

In health care settings the shifting of styles can take place a number of times within a consultation, and this is one marker of good practice. Consider this example:

> A practitioner has 20 minutes for a consultation, and he decides to spend the first 5–7 minutes using a *following style* with an anxious and distracted-looking elderly woman. The questions are open ended and give her time to tell a story about what has been going on. He deliberately slows down the pace of the consultation, and she calms down and becomes engaged in telling her story. The aim of his listening is to understand. He occasionally uses informing just to reinforce what she is saying. He is mostly saying such things as, "I see, you're worried about falling over" (listening), or "Tell me what exactly worries you about this medicine?" (asking).
>
> He then turns quite firmly to a *directing style*. He signals the shift by summarizing what she has said. "You are worried about the side effects of this medicine, and also whether you are taking the right dose as well. . . . " The patient feels understood, and this provides the practitioner with the opportunity to take his turn to be more actively involved. "I'd like to change direction now, and ask you some questions about your medicine use and its effect on you. Is that OK?" He then uses the skills of asking, listening, and informing to establish how best to make adjustments in the treatment and medication regimen. The questions are much more pointed, the information is clear and simple, and listening is used to clarify her understanding so that he can adjust the content and amount of information he provides. "What time of day do you take them?" "What have you noticed soon after you take them?" He provides advice and direction. "I'd like to suggest that you try this new medication, which is slightly stronger, but I don't believe that the side effects will get worse" (informing). "Yes, it's important that you take these tablets at the same time each day" (informing).
>
> Then there is a shift to a *guiding style*, because he wants to help her adapt to a new regimen of treatment and consider how she might cope at home. The purpose and content of the questions change, and the use of listening and informing reflect a conviction that motivation will be enhanced if as many solutions as possible come from her. "How do you see yourself succeeding this time?" "What's going to be the best regimen for you?" "What do you feel most confused about?" The other tools are also used. "Yes, that's right, and if your meals are more frequent, it

In health care settings the shifting of styles can take place a number of times within a consultation, and this is one marker of good practice.

might help" (informing), and "You are worried about the change, but you want to make it work" (listening). He summarizes the plan, and she agrees to return for a review.

A less flexible approach might affect outcome. If this practitioner had worked more rigidly within a directing style for most of the consultation and then turned to see what the patient thought and felt, engagement would have been undermined and commitment to change rendered much less likely. Flexible shifting among styles is a reflection of the desire to use your expertise effectively and to get the best out of the person you are serving.

Flexible shifting among styles is a reflection of the desire to use your expertise effectively and to get the best out of the person you are serving.

CONCLUSION

Patients seldom present with problems neatly wrapped up and responsive to a formulaic approach to communication. Asking, informing, and listening sound like rather simple tasks, perhaps not deserving of the label "skill." Compared with the complex things you need to be sure to get right in practice, these seem easy.

Yet these simple tasks can be done in very different ways and to different ends, and it becomes a highly skilled business to ask, listen, and inform in the right way to achieve your goals for the patient in the clinical situation. The precise choice of words, taken together with your body language, your use of silence, and the overall atmosphere of the consultation, can be a powerful tool. The way you communicate with patients can have a real effect not just on how they feel but on what they do and on their health outcomes. Your communication skills are themselves a treatment toolbox. The tools of asking, informing, and listening can be combined in a manner that is more or less efficient, effective, and skillful. How you use them depends on your purpose, and they can be used in different ways in the service of a directing, guiding, or following communication style.

The tools of asking, informing, and listening can be combined in a manner that is more or less efficient, effective, and skillful.

PART II

CORE SKILLS OF MOTIVATIONAL INTERVIEWING

CHAPTER 3

Practicing Motivational Interviewing

In this section, we present core skills of MI. These are not unfamiliar skills but, rather, are ones that you use in everyday practice. The difference is that these familiar skills are used in particular strategic ways in MI; they have a clear goal of health behavior change. The methods described here are for the particular (and common) situation in which the patient's path to optimal health calls for personal behavior change, a situation in which skillful guiding can be especially helpful and effective. As we discussed in the last chapter, particular forms of communication are appropriate for guiding, and in this part we devote a chapter to each of them.

A good guide will:

- *Ask* where the person wants to go and get to know him or her a bit.
- *Inform* the person about options and see what makes sense to them.
- *Listen* to and respect what the person wants to do and offer help accordingly.

As we explained in Chapter 1, the guiding style of MI works by enhancing patient commitment to change and adherence to treatment. Why does this happen? How can a relatively brief consultation trigger an enduring change in health behavior? A key to understanding this process is knowing the phenomenon of ambivalence.

AMBIVALENCE

People usually feel ambivalent about change. This is particularly so for change that is "good" for them in some way. Most people want to be healthy and are willing to do some things in the interest of their health. Most people are also comfortable with their familiar routines, and there are disadvantages to change. Some important health behaviors are unpleasant or even painful: lancing a finger for glucose monitoring, exercising after surgery, or enduring the ongoing side effects of adherence to a necessary treatment. Chances are that your patient already knows some good reasons for the behavior change that you have in mind, such as exercising more, quitting smoking, or eating healthier food. Chances are that your patient also *enjoys* the status quo—a sedentary lifestyle, smoking, or eating unhealthy food—and anticipates a downside to change. Conflicting motivations—to simultaneously want and not want—are normal and common. Consider the ambivalence in these patient statements:

> "I need to lose some weight, but I hate exercising."
> "I want to get up, but it hurts."
> "I should quit smoking, but I just can't seem to do it."
> "I mean to take my medicine, but I keep forgetting."

A telltale sign of ambivalence is the *but* in the middle.

People can and do get stuck in ambivalence. It is as if the arguments on either side of the *but* cancel each other out, and so nothing changes. Ambivalence is often experienced as first thinking of a reason to change, then thinking of a reason not to change, and then to stop thinking about it.

However, things can happen to move a person toward or away from behavior change. Your consultation with a patient can be one of these things. For some people, just receiving a diagnosis and a bit of advice can be enough to prompt significant changes in lifestyle. Often, however, patients go through a process of internal deliberation, conscious or not—a weighing of the pros and cons of behavior change. You can think of your patients as moving in one direction or the other during your health care consultations, as shown in Figure 3.1.

Perhaps your consultations sometimes seem to leave patients totally unmoved: "I've told him and told him, but he just won't change." How common this frustration is in health care! You explain over and over to patients what they need to do, how they could, why they should, and yet nothing happens. Remember the "righting reflex" discussed in Chapter 1? When you take a directing style with an am

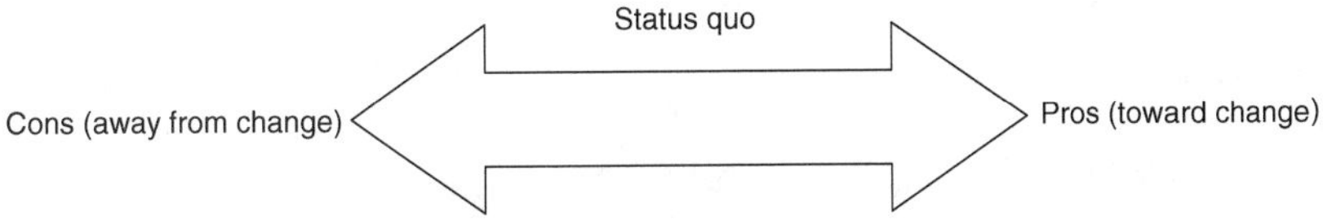

FIGURE 3.1. People can and do become stuck in ambivalence.

bivalent person, you are taking up one side of their own ambivalence—the pro-change side.

"Exercising and losing weight would decrease your risk of a heart attack."
"It's important for you to get out of bed and move around."
"I want you to stop smoking."
"This medicine won't help you if you don't take it faithfully."

A common patient response to these pro-change arguments is to fill in the other side of the ambivalence, to say, "Yes, but. . . ." When this happens, patients are making the arguments against change and literally talking themselves out of changing. What you want instead is for patients to talk themselves *into* changing, if it is compatible with their personal values and aspirations. In other words, your task is to elicit "change talk" rather than resistance from your patients.

LISTENING FOR CHANGE TALK

A first step in helping your patients make the arguments for change is being able to recognize change talk when you hear it. You already have an intuitive sense for it, learned from everyday social interaction.

Your task is to elicit "change talk" from your patients rather than resistance.

Suppose you are asking whether a friend will do something for you. There is a rich and well-developed vocabulary for this kind of negotiation, which is learned from life experience. Consider the following possible responses from your friend whom you have asked for a favor:

"Yes, I will."
"I might be able to."

"I wish I could."
"I'll try to get to it."
"I'll help if I can."
"I promise I'll do that for you tomorrow."
"I'll consider it."

What does each of these responses communicate? In particular, how likely is it that your friend will *actually* follow through on what you have asked? Each statement signals a different level of intention, and we understand its meaning from shared experience. These signals are also quite culture-specific. Someone from a different culture might well miss the subtleties and misunderstand what is being communicated.

Such communications are useful precisely because they actually do predict behavior. Not perfectly, to be sure. People may intentionally deceive you or for other reasons say what they think you want to hear, but within a relationship of goodwill and trust there is valuable information in such statements if you know what to listen for. By listening to what your patients say, you can tell how likely they are to change. Furthermore, when you hear change talk, you are doing it right. When you find yourself arguing for change and the patient defending status quo, you know you are off course.

When you hear change talk, you are doing it right. When you find yourself arguing for change and the patient defending status quo, you know you're off course.

So what exactly is change talk? When you are speaking with a patient about behavior change, there are six different themes you may hear, six different types of change talk. These are listed with examples in Table 3.1. Each type tells you something about the person's motivation.

Desire

The first theme of change talk is desire. Desire verbs include *want*, *like*, and *wish*. These tell you something that the person wants. These are desire statements:

"I *wish* I could lose some weight."
"I *want* to get rid of this pain."
"I *like* the idea of getting more exercise."

Desire statements tell you about the person's preferences either for change or for the status quo.

TABLE 3.1. Six Kinds of Change Talk

• *Desire*:	Statements about preference for change. "I *want* to . . . " "I would *like* to . . . " "I *wish* . . . "
• *Ability*:	Statements about capability. "I *could* . . . " "I *can* . . . " "I *might be able* to . . . "
• *Reasons*:	Specific arguments for change. "I would probably feel better if I . . . " "I need to have more energy to play with my kids."
• *Need*:	Statements about feeling obliged to change. "I *ought* to . . . " "I *have* to . . . " "I really *should* . . . "
• *Commitment*:	Statements about the likelihood of change. "I am *going* to . . . " "I *will* . . . " "I *intend* to . . . "
• *Taking steps*:	Statements about action taken. "I actually went out and . . . " "This week I started . . . "

Ability

A second type of change talk reveals what the person perceives as within his or her ability. The prototypical verb here is *can* and its conditional form, *could.*

> "I think I *can* come in twice a week."
> "I *could* probably take a walk before supper."
> "I might be *able* to cut down a bit."
> "I *can* imagine making this change."

Notice that ability-related change talk also signals motivational strength. "I definitely can" reflects much stronger confidence than "I probably could" or "I might be able."

Reasons

Change talk can express specific reasons for a certain change. There are no particular verbs here, although reasons can occur along with desire verbs.

"I'm sure I'd feel better if I exercised regularly."
"I want to be around to see my grandchildren grow up."
"This pain keeps me from playing the piano."
"Quitting smoking would be good for my health."

Need

Imperative language bespeaks a need or necessity. Marker verbs here include *need*, *have to*, *got to*, *should*, *ought*, and *must*.

"I *must* get some sleep."
"I've *got* to get back some energy."
"I really *need* to get more exercise."

Ambivalence often involves conflict among these four motivational themes: desire, ability, reasons, and need. In the following examples, the first phrase favors change, whereas the second phrase, separated by a *but*, favors the status quo:

"I really *should* [need] but I *can't* [ability].
"I *want* to [desire] but it hurts [reason]."
"I'd *like* to cut down my cholesterol [desire] but I do *love* eggs and cheese [desire]."

These first four kinds of change talk can be remembered by the acronym DARN—Desire, Ability, Reasons, and Need—and they have something in common. They are precommitment forms of change talk. They are leading in the direction of change, but by themselves they do not trigger behavior change.

To say "I want to" is not to say "I am going to."
To say "I can" is not the same as "I will."
To express reasons for change is not the same as agreeing to do it.
To say "I need to" is still not saying "I intend to."

For illustration, think of a person being sworn in as a witness in court*: "Do you swear to tell the truth, the whole truth, and nothing but the truth?" What is missing in the following answers?

* We thank Dr. Theresa Moyers for this example.

"I would like to [desire]."
"I could [ability]."
"It would help you if I did [reason]."
"I should [need]."

None of these is a satisfactory answer. What is missing is a fifth form of change talk.

Commitment

How does commitment sound? The quintessential verb here is *will*, but commitment has many forms. Some statements of strong commitment are:

"I *will.*"
"I *promise.*"
"I *guarantee.*"
"I *am ready* to."
"I *intend* to."

Do not miss lower levels of commitment, however, because they are also steps along the way. People signal an opening door with such statements as:

"I will *think* about it."
"I'll *consider it.*"
"I *plan* to."
"I *hope* to."
"I will *try* to."

These are meaningful statements to be encouraged. The latter two ("I *hope* to" or "I will *try* to") indicate a desire to change but signal that there is some doubt about the ability to do so. The language of conversations about change is rich with these signals.

Taking Steps

There is a sixth form of change talk you may encounter, particularly when you see patients repeatedly over time. These statements indicate that the person has taken, even if haltingly, some step toward change. He or she has done something that moves him or her in the direction of change:

"I tried a couple of days without drinking this week."
"I borrowed a book from the library about aerobic exercise."
"I bought some condoms."
"We went the whole month of February without eating any meat."
"I quit smoking for a week, but then started up again."
"I got one of those new test kits."
"I walked up the stairs today instead of taking the escalator."

Statements such as these can trigger some skepticism:

"Yes, but did you read it?" [the book on aerobics]
"Well, are you using them?" [the condoms]
"February—the shortest month!" [not eating meat]

What you should not miss is that actions such as these involve taking important tentative behavioral steps toward change, and such steps should be encouraged.

Do not worry about classifying change talk into the proper category. As you can see, there is some overlap. The same statement can contain two or more of these elements:

"I wish I could stop smoking [desire] because I'd have whiter teeth [reason]."
"I probably could lose ten pounds [ability] and I'd look better [reason]."
"I'll try [communicates some desire but uncertainty about ability]."
"I've got to do something to get my strength back, and I think I can [need, ability, and reason]."

The point is to attune your ears to change talk, to recognize and affirm it when you hear it.

How do these six forms of change talk fit together? The process begins with the precommitment types (DARN). People first talk about what they want to do (desire), why they would change (reasons), how they could do it (ability), and how important it is (need). When you evoke a patient's own desire, ability, reasons, and need for change, you are fueling the human engines of change. As DARN motivations are voiced, commitment gradually strengthens, and the person may take initial steps toward change. It is commitment and taking steps that predict durable behavior change. As indicated earlier, DARN statements in themselves may not trigger change, but they *do* presage the strengthening of commitment. Figure 3.2 shows how this looks.

It is worth noting here that when you explore DARN, you are

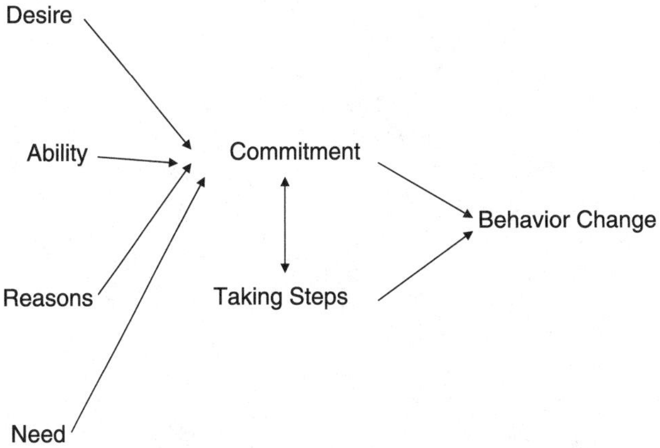

FIGURE 3.2. How change talk fits together.

touching on the patient's values and aspirations. When you hear DARN language, you are learning something about what your patients hope for, what matters to them. It gives you hints about more deeply held values. A patient who says, "I want to be there for my grandchildren" or "I don't want to be a burden to my family" is telling you something about the place of family in his or her priorities. These are important themes worth exploring a bit, rather than just letting them pass. The reason is that a deeply held value can be a powerful motivation for change. Help your patients talk about how a behavior change is consistent with what matters to them. When a behavior such as smoking truly collides with a more deeply held value, change can result. That is one reason that asking for DARN statements is a good idea.

> "Why would you *want* to quit smoking [desire]?"
> "How would you do it, if you decided to [ability]?"
> "What for you are the three best reasons for quitting [reasons]?"
> "How important is it for you to quit [need]?"

GUIDING THROUGH CHANGE TALK

Imagine an open meadow in a clearing surrounded by forest. In the meadow all manner of rich vegetation is growing. There is a carpet of green grasses, from which colorful wildflowers emerge. There are also clumps of green plants that in a garden might be regarded as weeds.

Your color vision allows you to differentiate the flowers from the carpet of green and from the clumps of weeds.

The carpet of grass is like the background of speech that you will hear from people when you listen. The person's own motivations for change are the flowers that pop up from the grass. The weeds are the person's arguments against change that, if encouraged, can choke out the flowers. The guiding style of MI is a process of gathering a bouquet. Because it is the patient who should be making the arguments for change, your task is to collect change talk. Each DARN change talk statement is like a flower. You collect these flowers into a bouquet that you periodically show to the patient, then continue to add to.

Here is another analogy: In successful MI, the change talk statements you collect from the patient are like little weights placed on the "pro-change" side of a balance. Helping patients to voice pro-change arguments gradually tips the balance in the direction of change.

This process of evoking change talk from the patient need not require a long time. You may be able to elicit significant change talk within the space of a few minutes of conversation. You also probably will have other chances when you see the patient for future consultations. Long-term health behavior change can emerge gradually over time with your successive guiding and encouragement. Success in evoking behavior change has more to do with your skill in the guiding style than with the length of time that you have to do it.

Listening for change talk offers another important benefit: It is how you learn to get better at guiding. Although we can give you some guidelines for using MI in practice, your real teachers are your patients. Whenever you try the guiding style, you get immediate feedback. If you hear more change talk, you know you're doing it right. When you seem to be eliciting arguments against change, your patient is telling you to try a different approach.

Although we can give you some guidelines for using MI, your real teachers are your patients. If you hear more change talk, you know you're doing it right.

CONCLUSION

So far we have summarized, in Chapter 1, the overall spirit of MI (collaboration, evocation, and honoring patient autonomy) and its basic principles, using the acronym RULE (Resist the righting reflex, Understand the patient's motivations, Listen to your patient, and Empower your patient). Chapter 2 placed MI within the context of a guiding style used naturally in everyday life. In this chapter we have explained the role of ambivalence and how to help patients get unstuck by listening for change talk. We outlined six types of change talk and how they fit together, leading to behavior change. In the next three chapters we return to the three core communication skills of asking, listening, and informing for a deeper look at how they can be used to help patients talk about, commit to, and undertake health behavior change.

CHAPTER 4

Asking

Asking seems simple enough. You pose a question and the patient responds. It's how you gather information. If only it were this straightforward!

This chapter is divided into two sections. The first deals with asking in general, and the second focuses on how asking is used in MI.

ASKING: SOME GENERAL CONSIDERATIONS

Diagnostic decision trees often require that you ask the *right* questions in order to make choices and recommendations. It is a familiar routine. Patients coming for health care expect you to ask a series of questions, some of which may be unexpected, as you deduce what is happening with their health. Asking a question places a demand on the other person to provide an answer. But the patient's expectation is that after you have finished asking all your questions, you will have the solution. This is especially true when you ask a series of *closed* questions, ones that elicit short answers such as "Yes" or "No" or a simple fact. With questions such as these, you are taking charge and implicitly taking responsibility to come up with the answer.

Closed Questions

Closed questions are an efficient way to gather specific information. The expected answer to a closed question is brief. Here are some examples:

"What is your address?"
"Where does it hurt?"
"Has your daughter had a fever?"
"How long have you been feeling dizzy?"
"Are the letters clearer with lens number one, or lens number two?"
"How often do you floss your teeth?"
"Have you been taking your medication?"
"When you do drink, how many drinks do you normally have?"
"Does it seem worse in the morning or in the evening?"

Open Questions

Open questions allow more room to respond. Whereas closed questions ask for specific information that the questioner regards as important, open questions invite responders to say what is important to them. Using open questions helps you understand what the person is experiencing and perceiving. Both closed and open questions elicit information. However, open questions often elicit more useful information than closed questions and also invite relationship.

"How are you feeling today?"
"Tell me from the beginning about how your pain developed."
"How can I help you?"
"How do you fit brushing and flossing into your daily routine?"

Asking even a few open questions and attending carefully to the person's responses can transform the quality of a health care consultation. Patients rightfully perceive open questions as showing personal interest and caring. When practitioners ask a few open questions and listen, patients tend to appreciate the amount of time the doctor spent with them and to be satisfied with the exchange. The skillful practitioner asking open questions appears to be taking lots of time yet can actually be making efficient progress.

The skillful practitioner asking open questions appears to be taking lots of time yet can actually be making efficient progress.

When you ask open questions, you give your patient more active involvement in and influence over the course of the consultation. Open questions also allow patients to tell you things that you have not asked about but that are potentially important. In addition, asking open questions can give you a chance to catch your breath, to stop, look, and listen in the midst of a busy day. The social etiquette of open questions is to make eye contact when asking them (rather than, for example, reading or writing in a chart) and to listen carefully to what the person has to say.

Open questions are those to which there is not an obvious short answer. They invite the person to offer their own experiences and perceptions. Here are some further examples:

"In what ways has this interfered with your life?"
"Tell me about a typical day when you drink."
"Tell me about your headache."
"Before we begin the exam, what are the things that concern you most today?"
"How are things going in your family?"
"What are you most worried about?"
"What are the things that you like and don't like about smoking?"
"This diagnosis must have been a shock. How are you dealing with it?"

Skillful Asking

Consider the difference between the two following consultations. In both of them, the practitioner is concerned that an elderly patient is not taking her medicines for asthma according to the prescription. Both rely on asking—the first through closed questions and the second with open questions.

Poor Practice: Relying on Closed Questions

The following begins with what we call a "spoiled" open question, evident later on as well—one that starts out open, but ends up closed.

Practitioner: Doctor, nurse.
Setting: Outpatient, primary care, or asthma clinic appointment.
Challenge: Brief review of medication use; to promote self-management.

PRACTITIONER: How are you getting on with the medicines? [open question] Have you been taking them regularly? [closed question]

PATIENT: I take them most of the time, and I feel OK except when I have an attack.

PRACTITIONER: The preventor inhaler is most important to take every day. Do you take that one regularly? [closed question]

PATIENT: Yes, most of the time.

PRACTITIONER: And what do you mean by most of the time? Is that every day, or do you miss days at a time, because that can be a problem. [closed question]

PATIENT: I wouldn't say that I miss many days, but it's not always so easy.

PRACTITIONER: You're on the high-dose regimen here, and it's important to take it every day, OK?

PATIENT: Yes, I know it's important, and I do try, honest I do.

PRACTITIONER: And what happens when you have your attacks [open question]? Does using your other inhaler help? [closed question]

PATIENT: Sort of. My husband gets scared.

PRACTITIONER: Well, it's good that you have him to help you like that. Will you remember to take your preventor inhaler every day, and not just the reliever when you have an attack? [closed question]

PATIENT: Yes.

The practitioner in this example was clearly capable of formulating useful open questions but managed to carelessly tag on it a closed question, which "spoiled" the value of the open question. A good illustration of this needless use of extra words is "And what happens when you have your attacks [open question]? Does using your other inhaler help [closed question]?" If the second question had been omitted, the first open question would have elicited how the inhaler was used and probably more information about other things, as well. Practitioners in training often make an interesting observation when reflecting on their use of closed questions: "Its exhausting, I feel rushed, and I always have to come up with the next question."

Better Practice: Carefully Chosen Short Open Questions

PRACTITIONER: How have you been doing? [open question]

PATIENT: Not too bad, thank you. I feel OK most the time, but when I have an attack it's different, you know.

PRACTITIONER: What happens? [open question]

PATIENT: Well, my husband gets really scared, and he yells at me to take my inhaler. He says that one of these days he's going to phone you up because he gets so scared.

PRACTITIONER: So what do you do then? [open question]

PATIENT: I use my reliever inhaler and things calm down, so I suppose we sort of manage, if you know what I mean. I'm not too worried, so I have to calm him down as well!

PRACTITIONER: And are you using the preventor inhaler? [closed question]

PATIENT: Yes, sort of.

PRACTITIONER: How are you getting on with it? [open question]

PATIENT: I don't really like it, to be honest, because I don't like the thought of taking all that steroid into my body. I get bruises from the steroid, which I find embarrassing. My hands look frightening and the bruises scare my grandchildren and my skin tears easily. But I know I should use it and my husband nags at me when I don't take it. You can imagine what goes on.

PRACTITIONER: And how can I be most helpful to you today? [open question]

PATIENT: Well, can you tell me what would happen if I didn't take the preventor in such high doses? Is it really essential, every day, to use the high dose? How about if I try the lower dose one if I guarantee to take it every day?

A number of qualities characterize skillful asking, many of which are apparent in the preceding example: The questions are short and the phrasing of them is simple; it feels to the patient as if it's a normal conversation connected to her experience. Important information (e.g., about the embarrassment at her bruised hands) is elicited via open questions, which do not necessarily have to extend the length of the consultation. Above all, open questions allow a practitioner to convey genuine interest in the patient. The practitioner in the first example might well have been interested in the patient, but poor communication skills prevented him or her from expressing this.

Most consultations, of course, call for both open and closed questions. A common approach is to build the exchange around initial key open questions, with closed questions being used only to funnel down and elicit specific information as necessary.

Some Useful Open Questions

If you need simply to obtain a few facts, such as whether certain symptoms have been experienced, then asking can be quite a simple matter. A few closed questions will suffice. Often health care is more complicated than that. Good open questions can serve multiple purposes. In addition to clarifying patients' symptoms, you might also want to know about their degree of discomfort, about their experience of something (e.g., pain relief), about their explanation for what happened (e.g., change in a child's condition), or about their concerns at quite a deeply personal level (e.g., after breaking bad news).

Here are a few examples of questions that cover multiple purposes, that are brief, and that, if accompanied by skillful listening (Chapter 5), can serve your purposes much more efficiently than asking a string of closed questions.

1. "*What's worrying you most today about this illness?*" This is a useful question for locating the patient at the center of the consultation. Responding respectfully to this concern will improve your rapport and provide a good platform for dealing with topics on your agenda.
2. "*What concerns you most about these medicines?*" If this patient is not taking her medicines properly and seems unhappy with them, a question like this will reveal a lot about her attitude, her behavior, and where the problem lies.
3. "*What exactly happens when you get that pain?*" Here, the door is open for the patient to tell a story. The use of the word *exactly* signals an intention to get to the bottom of the patient's concern. If you listen a while to the account, the answers to all sorts of factual and other questions may emerge.
4. "*What did you first notice about your child's condition?*" The word *notice* can be very useful. People usually respond well, because this word invites them to be the expert commentator about their experience of events and behavior. Information often comes flooding out, and they feel heard.
5. "*Tell me more about. . . .*"

An open question is an *invitation*. "May I ask you . . . ?" is a question that captures very well the polite and respectful quality of a service that is designed to meet the needs of the patient.

The Question–Answer Trap

It's easy to forget how anxious, bewildered, or preoccupied patients can be when they enter the consultation. Combine this with your own feeling of being tired or bored or going through a familiar routine, and the potential is there for a dysfunctional consultation. It can result in a pattern that we have called the question–answer trap.

Asking questions is easy; it can become routine, controlling, and overused to the exclusion of informing and particularly of listening. Your agenda predominates, and the patient can become a passive recipient of an investigation. It also sets you up to be the answer-giving expert. That can be quite appropriate in many forms of acute health care. However, as we shall see, when the subject is patient behavior change, a different and less directing style is needed.

One common manifestation of the question–answer trap in consultations about health behavior is the quantity–frequency investigation, which starts with "How much do you smoke?" and is followed by a family of questions such as "When did you start smoking?" and "Does your boyfriend smoke?" This approach tends to evoke resistance in the patient and frustration in the practitioner. It can feel like hard work because the onus is on you to think of the next question for the passive patient. Serial questions also tend to evoke defensiveness, often leading to answers that are half-truths as a means of protecting self-esteem.

Serial questions also tend to evoke defensiveness, often leading to answers that are half-truths as a means of protecting self-esteem.

In some circumstances, of course, you do need to ask many questions, and patients are often quite tolerant of this. If you do have a series of questions to ask, you can alert your patient beforehand, explaining that a rather question-ridden conversation is about to unfold, for particular reasons. This signals that the question–answer pattern is not your normal way of relating to people.

Routine Assessment: "Can I Just Ask You . . . ?" (Yawn)

One of us (Rollnick) went to a family physician with a distressing acute problem, and the consultation began thus: "How long ago did you stop smoking?" Asked the purpose of this question, the practitioner became slightly defensive and said with a wry smile: "It's not me who really wants to know, it's the computer!" This doctor was obliged to conduct routine assessments of lifestyle behaviors.

A familiar situation that can generate a stream of questions is the use of a standardized assessment form or intake procedure. There are usually good reasons for such procedures, but, when they are institutionalized, they can result in interviews that ignore the needs and concerns of the patient. When asked why patients in a diabetes clinic were stripped seminaked, weighed, and processed with questions *before* receiving any more conventional consultation, a service manager said, "Well, that's the way we have always done things around here." The familiarity of routine can cause one to overlook the social impact of the experience.

Even when routine questions are required, services can be designed to avoid institutionalized questioning as the dominant style in practice. When a standard questioning format is being used, one can still start in a natural manner with a series of open questions, acknowledging that some more specific questions will follow. The patient's responses to open questions often provide the answers to specific closed questions. Then you can use closed questions to fill in other needed information that did not emerge in response to the open questions.

There are more structured ways of avoiding what one practitioner called, perhaps unfairly, "death by assessment." One especially useful way of conducting a routine assessment is to use the "typical day" strategy as a framework for completing a form. Table 4.1 describes its use. Of course, with practice, the framework could be used at any point in a consultation when you want information, not just at the beginning. It can be used to ask about a "typical episode of pain," the "recent use of medication," or other things.

Summary

The ability to use asking thoughtfully and effectively is close to the heart of good quality patient care, whatever the problem being discussed and whatever communication style is being used. The tone, pacing, wording, and clarity of questioning, combined with a sense of curiosity and good listening, are some of the building blocks of quality communication. We turn now to how asking is used specifically within the guiding style of MI.

ASKING IN MI

> Carlos, a seasoned professional football coach, was in the park with his 4-year-old daughter. She fell over on her bicycle on the grass and burst into tears. He went down on one knee to comfort her, stayed in that position, and asked her a series of questions, waiting patiently for her to make up her mind each time.
>
> "Why did you fall over?"
>
> "I was going slow."
>
> "Yes, that's right, you went too slowly. And how could you go quicker?"
>
> "On the pavement."
>
> "And what could happen then?"
>
> "It would hurt if I fell over."

TABLE 4.1. Routine Assessment Using a "Typical Day"

Aims

To initiate an assessment that is lively and patient-centered in which many of your standard questions are answered. To have a normal conversation lasting 2–10 minutes in which rapport is enhanced, patients do most of the talking, and you learn a great deal about their personal and social context (including readiness to change). The formal assessment can be completed immediately afterward.

Principles

1. *Convey acceptance.* Do not pass judgment. Consider anything the patient says or does as acceptable, or at least as something that does not surprise you.
2. *Know your assessment schedule.* As the conversation unfolds, make a mental note of which areas of assessment are being covered and which are not.
3. *Fit the assessment into the interview, not the interview into the assessment.* It helps to place the paperwork aside, on the table.
4. *Stay curious.* Don't hesitate to interrupt with a request for help with more detail.
5. *Resist the investigative impulse.* Invading the patient's account with questions about problems can kill off the atmosphere of acceptance and curiosity.
6. *Focus on both behavior* ("What happened then?") *and feelings* ("When you closed the front door, heading for the shops, how were you feeling?").

Practice

1. *Acknowledge assessment and ask permission.* "I have a whole lot of questions on this form here, but I find it much easier to put this to one side and ask you to spend 5 to 10 minutes just taking me though a recent typical day in your life. I might go back to the form once we've done this to fill in the gaps; is that OK?"
2. *Locate a day.* "Can you think of a recent day that was fairly typical for you, an average sort of day?"
3. *Go through a "typical day."* Be mindful of time and the pacing. Slow it down if the patient runs too quickly through the story. Speed it up if you think it might take more than about 10 minutes.
4. *Check whether the patient wishes to add anything.* "Is there anything else about yesterday you want to say more about?"
5. *Ask any questions of your own.*
6. *Go back to your assessment to fill in the gaps, or do this later on.* Most patients do not mind your doing this after you have gone through a "typical day." In fact, if you remember to keep the form off your lap and avoid entering an investigative mode, many patients will actively help you complete the gaps quite willingly.
7. *Practice.* You know you are getting better when you interfere less and less with the "typical day" story. The patient's degree of comfort in telling the story is your indicator of success.

Note. Data from Rollnick, S., Mason, P., & Butler, C. (19990. *Health behavior change: A guide for practitioners*. Edinburgh: Churchill Livingston.

"So what do you feel like doing?"
"I am going on the pavement, bye, Papa . . . "

Carlos showed that the solutions should and could come from his daughter. He asked questions as Socrates did, leading his daughter to a solution. He created a supportive atmosphere, avoided the inclination to solve the problem for her, and elicited an informed choice by asking a series of *purposeful* questions. This is what we mean by asking in the service of a guiding style. It is one of the cornerstones of MI. It is an *invitation* to weigh the choices and to consider change. By asking such questions, you are evoking the person's own motivations, and by listening you come to understand the patient's perspectives—two of the core principles described in Chapter 2.

This is what we mean by asking in the service of guiding. . . . It is an invitation to weigh the choices and to consider change.

Agenda Setting

A good guide first finds out where the person wants to go. This can be particularly important in health care consultations, in which there may be many possible behavior changes that a patient could make to achieve better health. When there are multiple possible paths toward better health, who chooses what path to discuss?

We use "agenda setting" to refer to a brief discussion in which the patient is given as much decision-making freedom as possible. There might be topics that you are particularly concerned about, and a good guide will not hesitate to say what these are. But if you charge in, having decided about the topic yourself without consulting the patient, you lose an opportunity to learn what behavior change the patient is most ready to discuss. Consider the following example of a practitioner in a consultation about heart disease:

"OK, it sounds like you're doing well with the medication. Now can I ask you now about smoking? Any thought of giving it up?"

This is what we call the premature focus trap. The practitioner did not give the patient a chance to consider talking about other lifestyle changes.

In another form of premature focus, the practitioner, *within* a discussion about a specific behavior, focuses too soon on action. Let's assume that the patient in the preceding example *was* happy to talk about smoking. The practitioner's question, "Any thought of giving it up?"

The premature focus trap is sprung when the practitioner does not give the patient a chance to consider talking about other lifestyle changes. A second form of this trap occurs when the practitioner, within a discussion about a specific behavior, focuses too soon on action.

contains an immediate focus on a particular action, which might be premature for the patient, who is not all that ready. It might have been better to ask, "How do you feel about your smoking at this point?" This at least gives the patient a chance to get going and to feel comfortable talking about a difficult addiction.

Usually it is wise to start with understanding the patient's perspectives and preferences. Starting with patients' own concerns also tends to increase their willingness then to listen to yours. Often, as in the case of preventing or reversing disease, there is a menu of options to consider. Health-threatening behaviors tend to cluster in individuals. The patient might make healthful changes in diet, exercise, smoking, alcohol use, medication adherence, stress, anger, or social activities. Guiding questions, accompanied by listening, are a key to solving this problem.

Usually it is wise to start with understanding the patient's perspectives and preferences.

It is possible to provide a finite set of topics from among which patients can choose. One simple way to do this is with a "bubble sheet" that has a series of shapes, each containing one possible topic for conversation, including blank ones that the patient might like to fill in. In an outpatient cardiac clinic, for example, such a sheet might contain the bubbles shown in Figure 4.1, as well as a few empty bubbles (the ones with question marks in them).

Offering such a sheet, the practitioner can say, "If you like, we can talk about some changes you could make to improve your health. Here are some areas that can be important in controlling this illness that we could talk about, where people in your situation often consider changes. Are there any of these areas that you would like to talk about today? Or are there perhaps other things you want to raise that feel more important right now?"

This brief strategy usually takes a minute or so to complete, before you and the patient settle down to talk about an agreed focus for behavior change.

Then, after a few moments, it is usually feasible to mention those topics that you want to talk about, as well. Agenda setting is working well when the patient chooses one

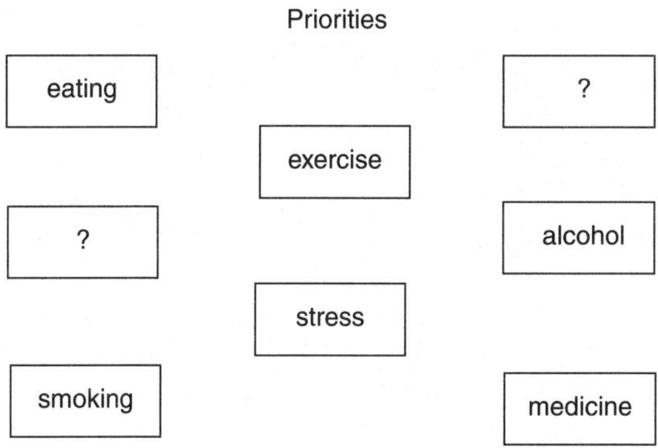

FIGURE 4.1. Sample agenda-setting sheet for use in a cardiac outpatient clinic.

topic about which you have a constructive conversation and when you have also aired your view about the topic. If your topic does not coincide with that chosen by the patient, a good general guideline is to start with the patient's priority. Agenda setting works well when the patient feels free to say, "No, thanks, not today."

This brief strategy usually takes a minute or so to complete, before you and the patient settle down to talk about an agreed focus for behavior change. With practice, you might not need a sheet of paper to guide you. Not every patient likes a visual aid. Agenda setting can be returned to at any point in the consultation if you get a bit lost or if you reach natural closure in discussing a particular change in behavior.

Agenda setting can be returned to at any point in the consultation if you get a bit lost or if you reach natural closure in discussing a particular change in behavior.

You might feel concerned that allowing patients to choose topics for discussion is risky because you are, after all, best placed to know which behaviors carry the greatest threats to health. Might you end up "letting the patient off the hook" by talking about something the patient chooses (e.g., exercise) but that you feel is less a problem than something else (e.g., smoking)? Many patients have been hearing the same talk about smoking over numerous years, with little benefit. If they make progress in one area, no matter how apparently unimportant, they might begin to learn the habit of success in a context in which failure is often the norm. Small successful steps in one area may lead to progress in another.

PRACTICAL SUGGESTIONS FOR ASKING THE RIGHT QUESTIONS

How do you decide which questions to ask in order to promote health behavior change? What question would be really helpful for this person? What will give a helpful perspective on his or her dilemma? What will elicit defensiveness versus change talk? It is a bit like finding the right path through a forest. Some paths lead in circles, go nowhere, or even lead one over the edge of a cliff; get it right and you can save a lot of time. Consider the difference between these two examples on the subject of diet:

Example 1: Policing "Bad" Behavior

PRACTITIONER: I need to ask you now, have you been keeping to the diet sheet you were given?

PATIENT: Yes, uhm, well, sometimes, but I forget, and its hard making separate meals from the rest of the family.

Example 2: A Helpful Guiding Question

PRACTITIONER: You're working on changing your diet. What would be most helpful for us to talk about today?

PATIENT: Its been really hard. I want to find meals that are good for me *and* the family, so that I don't have to make separate food for myself.

The first example has a policing tone to it, introduced by the closed question, which was in essence: "Have you been good?" Closed questions can elicit a feeling of being interrogated. The second consultation begins with an *invitation* in the form of an open question, giving the patient room to choose what to discuss. The question is delivered using a guiding style and helps the patient to take center stage. Change talk emerges right away.

How you respond to change talk is one of the core challenges in MI. In the preceding example, each of the four principles (RULE) discussed in Chapter 1 is relevant when considering what to say next. You would want to avoid the Righting reflex by not jumping in too soon with practical suggestions and to Understand this patient's motivations so as to elicit solutions from

The question was delivered in a guiding style and helped the patient to take center stage. Change talk emerged right away . . . How you respond to change talk is one of the core challenges in MI.

him or her. Listening might be the most productive next step (see Chapter 5), and you would want to Empower the patient by conveying a belief that change is possible and that together you can locate workable solutions.

The rest of this chapter focuses on providing some maps for locating useful guiding questions, which effectively open the door to change talk.

DARN!

One simple guideline is to ask open questions that can be answered with change talk. Remember the types of change talk discussed in Chapter 3? The DARN acronym can help you generate questions that elicit change talk.

- *Desire.* "What do you want, like, wish, hope, etc.?"
- *Ability.* "What is possible? What can or could you do? What are you able to do?"
- *Reasons.* "Why would you make this change? What would be some specific benefits? What risks would you like to decrease?"
- *Need.* "How important is this change? How much do you need to do it?"

Here are more generic questions about change, phrased to elicit all six types of change talk.

"Why might you want to make this change?" [desire]

"If you did decide to make this change, how would you do it?" [ability]

"What are the three most important benefits that you see in making this change?" [reasons]

"How important is it to you to make this change?" [need]

"What do you think you will do?" [commitment]

"What are you already doing to be healthy?" [taking steps]

One simple guideline is to ask open questions that can be answered with change talk.

Questions such as these tend to activate the patient toward change, eliciting his or her own motivations and creative ideas.

Each of these questions pulls for an answer that involves change talk. Questions such as these tend to activate the patient toward change, eliciting his or her own motivations and creative ideas. You do not really know the answer ahead of time, unlike Carlos, who led his daughter to a conclusion he clearly foresaw. For example, the most important reasons (benefits) that occur to you may not be the ones that most motivate the patient. The kinds of questions that frustrated practitioners sometimes want to ask elicit defensiveness:

"Why don't you want to ___________?"
"Why can't you ___________?"
"Why haven't you ______________?"
"Why do you need to ___________?"
"Why don't you ____________?"

The answer to each of these questions is a defense of the status quo. Ask people why they do not change and they will gladly tell you, and, in the process of telling, they reinforce the status quo.

The guiding questions that we present in this chapter are just examples. The underlying principle (Chapter 2) is to understand and explore the patient's own motivations for change. Our experience is that patients tend to move in healthy directions when offered this guiding style, much more so than when they are directed to do so.

Our experience is that patients tend to move in healthy directions when offered this guiding style, much more so than when they are directed to do so.

You know you are asking good guiding questions when some or all of these things happen:

- You feel connected with patients and interested in their answers.
- Your patients are talking about behavior change in a positive way.
- Your patients are wondering aloud about why and how they might change.
- A patient looks puzzled and engaged and is trying to work things out.
- A patient asks you questions about how or why he or she might change.
- Even when time is short, the consultation seems unhurried.

Using a Ruler

A ruler, or rating scale, from 1 to 10 can come in handy. These are already used in health care to ask for subjective ratings of, for example, the amount of pain a patient feels. Within MI, rulers have a dual purpose. They not only tell you about the patient's motivation but can also elicit change talk. A 1–10 ruler can be used to ask about various motivational dimensions, including readiness, desire, or commitment. Most patients are able to do this in a purely verbal form, although it is sometimes useful simply to draw a line on a piece of paper, place 0 and 10 at either end, and ask the patient to tell you where he or she is along this dimension.

Rulers not only tell you about the patient's motivation but can also elicit change talk.

For example, you can take the first step by asking such questions as:

> "How strongly do you feel about wanting to get more exercise? On a scale from 1 to 10, where 1 is 'not at all,' and 10 is 'very much,' where would you place yourself now?"
>
> "How ready do you feel to make this change? On a scale from 1 to 10, where 1 is 'not at all ready,' and 10 is 'completely ready,' where would you place yourself now?"
>
> "How important would you say it is for you to stop smoking? On a scale from 1 to 10, where 1 is 'not at all important,' and 10 is 'extremely important,' what would you say?"

A second step is to ask the patient why he or she has given you one particular number, say 5, and not a lower number. The answer to this question is change talk, and you are now able to explore this in some detail. Another useful variation is to ask what would have to happen to make the chosen number go up. But beware—frustration or the righting reflex might lead you to ask the opposite question: "Why are you at 5 and not 10?" The answer to that question is defense of the status quo.

One other warning about using rulers: They are only as good as the quality of rapport between you and the patient. If you launch into this assessment in an investigative manner, too soon, without genuinely wanting to understand and encourage the patient, you might well elicit a defensive rating of some kind. "Oh, yes, I'm very ready to stop smoking . . . " might come from a patient who is really just telling you what she or he thinks you want to hear. The fact that you are using a ruler does not mean that the answers are always reliable. Good rapport and the use of a guiding style can help enormously to improve the reliability of the exercise.

Some practitioners and services keep a record of the results of this kind of assessment. You might find this particularly useful when you see the same patient again, just to remind you (and the patient) about how things might have changed.

Assessing Importance and Confidence

Among the most productive questions are two simple ones about the importance of change to the patient and his or her confidence in succeeding. Here the ruler can be very useful. The goal is to use these questions as a platform for developing understanding and for eliciting change talk and to make sure that you efficiently focus your energies on the area of greatest need. If your inquiry is a genuinely curious one, and if your rapport with the patient is good, a patient's own motivations arise in the conversation with ease.

Among the most productive questions are two simple ones about the importance of change to the patient and his or her confidence in succeeding. Here the ruler can be very useful.

The first step is to ask about the importance of change and then, if it seems appropriate, to elicit a numerical rating. "How important is it for you to ____? Could you tell me, on a scale from 1 to 10, where 1 is 'not at all important,' and 10 is 'extremely important,' how important is it for you to __________?" Ask 100 overweight patients this question about weight loss, and you'll get numbers all along the scale, but mostly between 3 and 7. The second step, just like that mentioned earlier, is to ask: "Why did you give yourself a score of ____ and not 1?" The answer to this question will be the reasons that the patient sees the change as important (i.e., change talk). You learn not only how important the change is subjectively but also *why* it is important to the patient.

If your inquiry is a genuinely curious one, and if your rapport with the patient is good, his or her own motivations arise in the conversation with ease.

The same questions can be asked about confidence in his or her ability to change: "On a scale from 1 to 10, where 1 is 'I'm certain that I could not,' and 10 is 'I'm certain that I could,' how confident are you that you could __________ if you decided to? What number would you give yourself right now?" Then, after getting the rating, you ask, "And why did you give yourself a ____ and not 1?" Here, the basis for the patient's confidence in his or her ability to change will be expressed. It can also be helpful to look up the scale and ask questions such as "What would help you to get a higher score?" or "How can I help you to move higher up the scale?"

Patients can need different kinds of help from you depending on their ratings on these two scales. Consider these two patients: Both lie somewhere around the midpoint of a readiness-to-change continuum;

both express ambivalence and reluctance to quit smoking; but they have very different underlying motivations.

> Smoker A: "Here I am, 55 years old, and I'm diagnosed with emphysema. I really need to quit smoking, but how? I've tried so many times and failed. It just seems pointless to try." [Importance: 9 Confidence: 2]
>
> Smoker B: "Sure, I know you think it's bad for me, and in the long run it probably is, but smoking is part of my social life. I tell you, I've been in international competition as an athlete, and if I decide to do something, I know I can succeed. This just isn't a priority for me right now." [Importance: 2 Confidence: 9]

Patients who are high on importance but low on confidence, like Smoker A, need encouragement that change is possible and some specific ideas about how to do it. They are quite different from patients who are high on confidence but low on importance, such as Smoker B. If you talked about the *why* of change (importance) with Smoker A, and the *how* of change (confidence) with Smoker B, you would probably be wasting your time, because these are not the areas in which they need your help. Assessing your patients on these dimensions allows you to use the precious time you have in the consultation in a way that is most congruent with their greatest need. If the major obstacle to change is low importance, using these questions will allow you to understand that and efficiently address the issue of importance. The same is true for confidence. Far from adding to the length of consultations, substituting this kind of approach for a "one size fits all" style of intervention allows greater efficiency and patient engagement, with added opportunities for eliciting change talk.

> *Assessing your patients on importance and confidence in their ability to change allows you to use the precious time you have in the consultation in a way that is most congruent with their greatest need.*

Pros and Cons

Asking about the pros and cons provides you with a set of key guiding questions that are particularly useful if someone seems uncertain about change. This gives you the opportunity to explore ambivalence. It gives the patient time to come face-to-face with uncertainty in an accepting atmosphere in which his or her inner motivations are free to surface. This lies at the heart of MI.

First, ask your patient what is good about the way things are now. Asking this gives you some momentum to ask about the not-so-good things about the status quo. These two general questions can be applied to any change topic. Notice that the first question elicits arguments for not changing, and the second elicits change talk. The most common effect of asking either one of these questions is that the patient will present you with both sides of his or her ambivalence.

Asking about the pros and cons provides you with a set of key guiding questions that are particularly useful if someone seems uncertain about change.

With regard to smoking, the first question might be: "What do you like about smoking?" Note that this question is asked without any shade of disapproval or sarcasm. If your voice tone implies "What could you *possibly* like about smoking?" you will elicit defensiveness. The question is asked with honest interest and curiosity about the perceived benefits of continuing to smoke. Once you have elicited the patient's perceptions of the good aspects of the behavior, you can follow up with a second question. For example, "And what's the downside for you? What are the not-so-good things about smoking?"

A useful way to conclude this conversation is for you to summarize briefly your understanding of the patient's account of pros and cons of the behavior as he or she sees it, using his or her own words whenever possible. Asking a key question such as "Where does this leave you now?" often provides patients with an invitation to take things a step further, to be in the driver's seat of change in their lives.

Key Questions: What Next?

A "key question" is one that tests the patient's level of commitment to change. A key question is a good follow-up after any of the preceding discussions: DARN motivations, rulers, importance and confidence, or pros and cons. The essence of a key question is "What next?" Here are some examples of key questions:

"So what do you make of all of this now?"
"So what are you thinking about smoking at this point?"
"What do you think you'll do?"
"What would be a first step for you?"
"What, if anything, do you plan to do?"
"What do you intend to do?"

Notice that the normal answer to any of these questions would be commitment language. The strength of commitment expressed by the patient gives you a read on how likely the change is to happen. Low commitment suggests a need for further exploration of DARN themes in this or a subsequent visit.

As a patient expresses some intention to change, it can be useful to get more specific. *When* will the patient make or begin this change? Exactly *what* will the patient do? *How* will the patient succeed? Research shows that people are much more likely to carry through with behavior change when they express their intentions in more specific terms of what, when, and how. But do not press for a commitment that the patient is not ready to make. The question is, what is the person ready, willing, and able to do now?

Using Hypotheticals

For patients who are less ready to change, it is less threatening if you take one step back with them and talk in hypothetical language. This allows them greater freedom to envision change. Here are some guiding open questions phrased in hypothetical language:

"What might it take for you to make a decision to ______?"
"If you did make a change in __________, what might be some of the benefits?"
"Suppose that you did decide to _____________. How would you go about it in order to succeed?"
"Let's imagine for a moment that you did ____________. How would your life be different?"
"What would it take for you to go from a 5 to an 8 [on importance]?"
"How would you like things to be different?"
"Suppose you continue on without making any change in __________. What do you think might happen in 5 years?"

For patients who are less ready to change, it is less threatening if you take one step back with them and talk in hypothetical language.

Imaginative leaps are also possible if you have good rapport with the patient and if she or he is clearly comfortable with the discussion. Consider the use of this kind of question:

"What currently impossible thing, if it were possible, might change everything?"
"If you were in my shoes, what advice would you give yourself about_______?"

"How has [this behavior] kept you from growing, from moving forward?"

"What do you most want to be happening in your life a year from now, 5 years, or even 10 years down the road?"

CONCLUSION

This chapter has outlined the use of questions both in general and in the service of a guiding style. When it comes to the latter, taking your time often leads to faster progress. Consultations about behavior change call for this attitude. A few well-spent minutes can sow the seeds for change later on. Many practitioners have had the experience of a returning patient saying something like: "There was one thing you said that made all the difference. . . ." At the heart of your use of MI is a conviction that patients have most of the answers within them. Once you enter this frame of mind, the right questions usually follow.

CHAPTER 5

Listening

Long before there was any scientific basis for health care, there were healers who had learned to listen carefully. There is something about being heard and understood, about being the focus of full compassionate attention, that is in itself healing. Such listening is, we believe, one reason why patients so frequently seek out and appreciate the services of alternative healers and those health care practitioners who listen well. Although some people seem to have an almost innate talent for listening, the outcome of our research efforts matches our experiences in training: You can become more skilled and efficient with this tool, and it makes a difference to the outcome of the consultation and beyond.

This chapter takes you through the skill of listening in some depth. We begin with some general considerations and then turn to the use of listening within a guiding style, a skill that lies at the heart of MI.

THE CASE FOR LISTENING

To be sure, the pressures of practice can discourage taking such apparently "unproductive" time. Yet there are some good reasons to hone your listening skills.

- Listening helps you to gather important information that you might otherwise miss.
- Even a little high-quality listening can greatly promote your relationship with a patient. It can take as little as 1–2 minutes. Long after

the specifics have faded, patients often remember that nurse, doctor, or social worker who really listened to them.

- Patients whose providers listen to them are more comfortable and satisfied with their care, more likely to be open and honest, and, we believe, more likely to adhere to advice.
- When you take time to listen, *patients feel as though you've spent a longer time with them than you actually have.* On the other hand, a consultation that is limited to asking and informing often feels shorter than it really is; patients tend to underestimate how much time you spent with them.
- Perhaps most important, there is something very helpful about good listening itself. You may have the impression that you are "not doing anything," but good listening is a large component of those important "nonspecific" aspects of healing. Just listening can foster change.

When you take time to listen, patients feel as though that you've spent a longer time with them than you actually have.

Listening can save you time, because you develop an ability to quite quickly grasp the essence of the patient's concerns. This allows you to move on to another topic more easily.

Beneath all the technical aspects covered in this chapter is a simple notion: Listening involves an attitude of curiosity and acceptance of the patient while you are engaged in this process. The more skilled you become, the easier you will find it to integrate brief episodes of listening into routine practice. This can save you time, because you develop an ability to quickly grasp the essence of the patient's concerns. This allows you to move on to another topic more easily.

LISTENING: SOME GENERAL CONSIDERATIONS

A practitioner who is listening, even if it is for just a minute, has no other immediate agenda than to understand the other person's perspective and experience. There is no intent to intervene or fix things. The practitioner is simply present with the person, open to whatever he or she is experiencing and wishes to say.

A practitioner who is listening, even if it is for just a minute, has no other immediate agenda than to understand the other person's perspective and experience.

When might you use listening? Quite simply, at any point in the consultation. It can and should be integrated into routine practice and form a normal part of whatever assessment, diagnostic, or management task you are carrying out. It is a tool that can be used very effectively in the service of a directing style, combined with asking and informing. Here are some key situations for use of listening:

• *The first part of a consultation.* In fact, it's risky *not* to listen at the start of consultation. Interrupt this activity and you can sow the seeds of dysfunction quite rapidly. The patient might withdraw, become frustrated, or bring you back to the concerns that you ignored in the first place. Often patients have plucked up some considerable courage to come for a health care appointment and to tell their story to their practitioner. One of the commonest patient criticisms of consultations is not being allowed to tell this story. An early interruption sets the scene for a developing sense of not being heard.

• *Brief episodes throughout the consultation.* Patients signal the need for this when they seem confused, anxious, disengaged, upset, or annoyed. For your part, when you are not sure about a diagnostic or management matter, listening is a powerful way of unraveling what is going on.

• *After you ask an open question.* It is an invitation to the patient to speak, and your opportunity to listen and understand.

There are other situations in which a directing style can be put to one side and a following style is called for, in which listening is paramount. Here are some specific examples.

- You walk into the examining room, and the patient says, "I have just had a terrible experience this morning."
- You have had to break some bad news to a patient, and now it is time to let him or her absorb it and respond.
- You sit down at the bedside of a dying patient who is just awakening. He or she smiles and says "Hello." There is nothing that you need to ask or do immediately.

There are times when the most important and the most healing thing you can do is simply to be there with your patients, to take the time to listen and understand. Here you would use a following style. You might provide information and ask questions, but your primary purpose is to *follow* the needs of the patient—for example, when breaking bad news or when talking to someone who is particularly distressed or anxious.

The next sections discuss some practicalities of listening in health care. We explore some uses of listening, provide some tips, and touch on some pitfalls to avoid.

Opening the Door

You open the door to listening by extending an invitation. Most often this takes the form of an open question, accompanied by signals that you intend to listen. "How are you?" has become a superficial greeting, offered in passing without the expectation that the other will actually elaborate. What, then, distinguishes a disingenuous "How are you?" from a real invitation to talk and be heard? How do we tell the difference in normal conversation?

Two key signals are eye contact and lack of distraction. Consider the differences in the meaning of "How are you?" when asked by:

- A person while passing in the hallway without pausing or making eye contact.
- A nurse who is paging through a medical chart and readying a blood pressure cuff.
- A physician who walks into the examining room, makes eye contact, smiles, sets aside whatever she or he is carrying, and pulls up a chair.

The latter is communicating not only verbally ("How are you?") but also nonverbally that right at the moment listening is the most important thing on the agenda. These nonverbal cues are even more important than the words of invitation. One commonly used training exercise requires a speaker to talk about a topic on which he or she can continue for some time with minimal support from the listener. The listener's task is the harder one: to communicate to the speaker that he or she is listening, hearing, and understanding *but without speaking a word* or even making vocal sounds, such as "uh huh." The listener has only nonverbal cues to communicate listening and understanding, such as eye contact, facial expression, head movement, and so on.

The verbal part of the invitation to be listened to is a simple opening. Here are a few examples:

PATIENT: I just had a terrible experience this morning.

PRACTITIONER: Tell me about it.

PRACTITIONER: (*coming bedside*) Hello, how are you feeling this evening?

PRACTITIONER: (*entering the consulting room*) Good morning! Tell me what's on your mind today.

PRACTITIONER: (*with some standard questions to ask*) In a little while I'll need to get some specific information from you, but before we do that, let me just take a few minutes to hear about what made you decide to come here today.

Asking Is Not Listening

What is a good listener? After you open the door with an invitation and are paying attention, what should you do next?

Many people confuse listening with asking questions, but these are two different communication tools. A question places a demand on the person to give you an answer. A question also points the person in a particular direction, putting the spotlight on one particular topic or area that is of interest to the questioner. The psychologist Thomas Gordon called questions "roadblocks" to listening. For the person to continue down the road they were on before the question, they have to deal with the roadblock, go around it, and then get back on the path. Ask two or three questions in a row, and surely the person is derailed from his or her original course. You are the one who is in charge, not the speaker. That is not necessarily a bad thing; asking is also part of your job. If someone is acutely ill and you need to make a diagnosis by working your way through a mental decision tree, you probably need to ask a series of questions. But for pure listening, the only question you need is an opening invitation.

Asking and listening are not the same thing.

Silence

Silence is often a good teacher. If you are silent, even for a brief moment, you are not voicing all of the roadblocks that people normally throw in each other's way: agreeing, disagreeing, instructing, questioning, warning, reasoning, sympathizing, arguing, suggesting, analyzing, persuading, approving, shaming, reassuring, interpreting, and so on. Silencing these spoken roadblocks is a good start toward real listening.

Roadblocks to listening include agreeing, disagreeing, instructing, questioning, warning, reasoning, sympathizing, arguing, suggesting, analyzing, persuading, approving, shaming, reassuring, and interpreting.

A next step is to silence your inner chatter and focus full attention on understanding the person who is with you. Even without voicing the roadblocks, you may be *thinking* them. How easy it is, while seeming to listen, to be thinking ahead to what you need to do next! To fully listen, even that inner chatter is hushed, and you give your full attention to listening, hearing, and understanding. Here's a new meaning for *attending* physician!

Even without voicing the roadblocks, you may be thinking them. . . . To fully listen, even that inner chatter is hushed.

Facilitative Responses

Pure silence can also make some people uneasy. Despite your best nonverbal attending, if you say absolutely nothing, some patients will start to wonder what you are thinking or whether you are actually listening at all. A simple step is to reengage the vocal cords a bit and offer a few small facilitative responses as simple as "mm hmm," or "I see," or "say some more about that." Of course, responses such as these could be programmed into a computer, and thus they are not proof positive that you are listening.

Proof positive that you are listening, hearing, and understanding is to reflect back to the person a short summary of how you understand what he or she said. Parrots cannot do this—it involves more than repeating.

In Somewhat Different Words: Listening by Reflecting

Proof positive that you are listening, hearing, and understanding is to reflect back to the person a short summary of how you understand what he or she said. Parrots cannot do this—it involves more than repeating. We have also found that actors cannot do this without special training. Actors are perfectly good at being silent, attending, and giving facilitative responses, but reflective listening is a skill that takes special practice. Actors can on demand *look like* they are listening, but the real thing is more challenging.

So what is the real thing? Let's start with an example in which the practitioner, after asking an open question, and for purely illustrative purposes, does absolutely nothing but reflective listening:

PRACTITIONER [social worker, doctor, psychologist, dietician, nurse, physical therapist, counselor]: We're coming toward the end of our session, but you said quite quickly a moment ago that there was something that made you feel not quite right.

PATIENT: Well, yes, I haven't been feeling that great. It started about a month or two back, and at first I thought I was just imagining it, possibly because I was working so hard and hadn't been exercising much, you know what I mean?

PRACTITIONER: You're working a lot and haven't been feeling quite right.

PATIENT: Well, I thought it was just that, but then I sort of felt tired and weak when I had any kind of exertion, like I was short of breath, and I have never had that before. Not even when I have been out of shape. Even walking up the stairs at home, I notice it.

PRACTITIONER: That's definitely unusual for you.

PATIENT: Yes, that's right, on the stairs, but also sometimes when I was just sitting down not actually doing much. At first I thought it was the stress. Now I wonder if it's my lungs or heart.

PRACTITIONER: You're not 100% sure what's going on, and it's got you a little scared.

PATIENT: Yes, it's been sort of creeping up on me, I mean I'm usually the rock of the family, and even at work, but now this.

PRACTITIONER: You're used to being in charge.

PATIENT: Not necessarily in charge, but reliable, you know? But I think it's beginning to get too much for me, and I feel like things are getting out of control.

PRACTITIONER: Like there's not enough time to look after yourself.

PATIENT: That's exactly right. I have to sort this out.

PRACTITIONER: You want to know what's going on and do something about it.

PATIENT: Well, this is the first step, I said to myself, I want to mention this to you.

Each reflection is a short summary of what is happening at that moment.

What is going on here? This practitioner is being a very active partner in the communication process and is taking a minute or two to understand the patient's own perceptions and concerns. In order to do this kind of listening, the practitioner must attend to the patient, hear the words accurately, and then form a hypothesis about (literally reflect on) what the patient means so as to be able to say it back in somewhat different words. The practitioner reflects those "different words" back to the patient, and then something interesting happens. The patient either confirms or disconfirms the practitioner's hypothesis. The patient either says, in essence, "Yes, that's right" and continues to elaborate, or "No, that's not quite right" and continues to elaborate. There's no penalty for guessing wrong here. Either way the patient is likely to tell you as long as you reflect in somewhat different words. Even direct ion can have this effect sometimes, but usually parroting falls flat in short order. Sometimes a reflection takes the form of "continuing the paragraph," anticipating what the patient might say next but that is yet unsaid.

Sound complicated? It is; it takes practice. The good news is that it's a learnable skill, and one that is clinically quite useful. Furthermore, your patients are your teachers. Each time you try a reflection, you get immediate feedback about its accuracy, and so over time you get better at it.

The practitioner forms a hypothesis about what the patient means so as to be able to say it back in somewhat different words . . . and then something interesting happens. The patient either confirms or disconfirms the hypothesis.

Here is a somewhat longer consultation in which, again, *just for purposes of illustration*, the practitioner again uses only reflective listening. If you enjoy a challenge, cover the page with a sheet of paper and reveal one line at a time. For each patient response, before you look at what the practitioner says next, consider how you might reflect what the patient has said.

Your patients are your teachers. Each time you try a reflection, you get immediate feedback about its accuracy, and so over time you get better at it.

A patient in the hospital needs to decide whether or not to have an operation, and your colleague is frustrated because she cannot get a clear answer from him. "Every time I ask him, he just breaks down weeping. Could you talk with him?"

PRACTITIONER: [psychologist, social worker, nurse, doctor, counselor]: You said you were worried about your possible operation.

PATIENT: *Worried* is not the word, it's so complicated I don't know where to begin.

PRACTITIONER: And it's causing you quite a lot of distress. [continuing the paragraph]

PATIENT: Last night I hardly slept, I was so worried. (*Begins to weep.*)

PRACTITIONER: (*Stays silent, hands him a tissue.*) It's like things are coming to a head.

PATIENT: It's not like me to cry like this.

PRACTITIONER: This is really important.

PATIENT: This is the big one. (*Continues to weep.*)

PRACTITIONER: It feels like a big decision that you have to make, one way or another.

PATIENT: That's right, as every day goes by I get closer and closer to having to decide.

PRACTITIONER: But not much clearer. [again continuing the paragraph with a guess]

PATIENT: That's the problem, because if have the operation, I know I might not last long afterward. It's a big risk. That's what I've been told, as simple as that.

PRACTITIONER: And if you don't have the operation, it's not that easy either.

PATIENT: Well, not exactly, it's a question of time, you see. They say I might have just a few months left, and all I know for sure is that I want to be there for my family.

PRACTITIONER: That's the most important thing for you right now.

PATIENT: You should see my son (*laughs*), he says I'm still the same old rude rascal, nothing's changed, even though I am supposed to be so ill.

PRACTITIONER: Sometimes you almost feel back to normal.

PATIENT: When I'm with him, its great, but then, there's no escaping this, really.

PRACTITIONER: You feel trapped.

PATIENT: Yes, that's it, I lie here and think about taking the chance and having the operation, then I imagine it going badly, then I try to stop thinking about it.

PRACTITIONER: You're just not sure what to do.

PATIENT: Sometimes I think that, well, you people do these operations, and I should put my trust in you.

PRACTITIONER: If you had the operation and it worked out well, that would be a good outcome.

PATIENT: I think I'll probably go along with this, but I just need some time to get used to the idea, and then I'll let you know.

PRACTITIONER: You need some time to work through this decision about the operation.

PATIENT: I will decide soon.

PRACTITIONER: (*offering a little longer summary of what has been said*) Let me see if I understand what you've been telling me, and do let me know if I've missed anything. This decision is not an easy one for anyone to make. Whichever way you go, there's a risk that you might not be there for your family. You've been told that without the operation you have only a few months, but the operation is also risky. You're getting closer to making the decision, though, and you just need more time to think it over. You feel especially good when you see your family, and you are thinking as much about them as you are about yourself.

PATIENT: Yeah, that's quite right, I don't really need any more information, and this isn't a decision you can make for me. It's just good to talk this through with you.

Note a few things about the reflections in this example. First, they are all *statements* rather than questions. The practitioner is not asking, "Is this what you mean?" If you were listening to an audiotape, you would also hear that the practitioner's voice inflection turns *down* at the end of a good reflection and not *up* as when asking a question. This can feel odd at first, but only to you, not to the patient. Offering reflections as statements rather than questions makes patients more comfortable, and they keep talking. A patient is more likely to elaborate if you say:

The practitioner's voice inflection turns down at the end of a good reflection, and not up as when asking a question.

"You're feeling anxious about this." [voice inflected down at the end]
rather than:
"You're feeling anxious about this?"[voice inflected up at the end]

Also note that the practitioner's skillful responses in the above example sometimes reflected content that the patient had not actually said but that *might* be what the patient meant or was thinking. Reflections need not be restricted to what the person has said directly. Sometimes you are continuing the paragraph by offering what the next as-yet-unsaid sentence might be rather than just repeating the one that has gone before.

The Skill of the Summary

In the final response of the preceding case example, the practitioner collected the main themes that the patient had offered and pulled them together in a summary. In a way, each reflection is a short summary of what is happening at that moment, but this kind of collecting summary looks back over part or all of the conversation and offers an abstract. There is skill to knowing what to include in such a summary. Later on in this chapter we give you some specific guidelines for choosing what to include in summaries when listening is used in MI. Here, however, the practitioner just attempted to pick up the main themes that the patient had raised.

Offering reflections as statements rather than questions makes patients more comfortable, and they keep talking.

Summaries can serve several very useful functions:

- A good summary shows in a powerful way that you have been listening carefully to and remembering what the patient said. This is in itself a positive message that can strengthen your working relationship.
- Giving a summary causes you to draw together the pieces of the picture and to see whether you have missed something important. To do this, you can follow a summary by asking "What else?"
- A summary allows you to reemphasize certain aspects of what the patient has said by including and highlighting these themes. This aspect of summaries is particularly useful within the guiding style.
- A summary frees you to change direction. It is a gentle and positive way to draw your period of listening to a close and move on to the next task.

Asking and Listening

Although they do represent two different tools of communication, asking and listening fit naturally together and complement each other. A therapeutic approach known as client-centered or person-centered counseling, introduced by psychologist Carl Rogers, relies primarily on a skillful combination of asking and listening. This is also a natural combination to use in health care.

For most people, asking questions is much easier than reflecting. As a result, even when practitioners try to be good listeners, it is common for them to ask a series of questions in a row with little or no reflective listening in between.

We offer three practical recommendations about questions *while you are listening.*

1. Try to ask open rather than closed questions.
2. Try not to ask two questions in a row.
3. Try to offer at least two reflections for every question you ask.

A resulting rhythm would be an open question followed by reflective listening to what the patient offers. For example:

PRACTITIONER [nurse, doctor, podiatrist]: So you've been having quite a bit of pain in your feet. Tell me about that.

PATIENT: Sometimes it hurts so much that I have trouble walking. I have to go up and down stairs at work, and that's really hard.

PRACTITIONER: And that pain is fairly constant, every day. [reflection, a guess]

PATIENT: Just about, yes. Less on the weekends when I'm not working.

PRACTITIONER: There's something different about the weekends. [reflection]

PATIENT: Well, like I said, I'm not at work, and I stay home more.

PRACTITIONER: What kind of shoes do you wear on the weekend? [closed question]

PATIENT: I usually wear bedroom slippers or go barefoot around the house.

PRACTITIONER: And that feels better. [reflection]

PATIENT: My feet still hurt, but not as much. But if I go out on Saturday night, then I wear spikes.

PRACTITIONER: High heels—higher than you wear to work. [reflection]

PATIENT: A little maybe, but I wear heels at work, too.

While you are listening, try to offer at least two reflections for every question you ask.

Some Concerns about Listening

It is hard to do harm with good listening, in which a sense of genuine warmth and curiosity is present. If your reflections are too similar to what the person said, if there is too much a straight repetition, you can go around in circles.

However, there can be a downside to listening that you will quickly discover. Most people experience so little good-quality listening in their lives that they are quite hungry for it. When they meet someone who actually takes the time to listen, hear, and understand, it is such a rewarding experience that they could literally talk for hours. That, we find, is a great worry among practitioners about listening to their patients. It is an understandable worry, but one that is actually quite manageable. Most practitioners already know good and gentle ways to bring a consultation to an end when it is time to move on. A closing summary is just one of these. The truth also works: "Thank you for sharing this with me. What you have told me today has really helped me get a much better understanding of the situation. I wish I could listen longer, but I have to see someone else now, and I don't like to keep people waiting. Let's talk more about this the next time I see you."

Some practitioners also worry that if they pull the cork out of the bottle, it will overflow: "If I listen to my patients in this way, will they fall apart right there in my consulting room? After all, I'm not a psychologist." And, again, time is often a concern. It certainly can happen that when a compassionate listener takes even a little time to understand, the person can be moved to tears. It's a question of balance. No one would endorse not listening to patients; nor could you justify losing control of the time and of other tasks that you need to carry out. Patients also do not necessarily want to experience their fear, anger, sadness, or frustration in large doses.

Effective and gentle ways of bringing listening to a close:

- *Summarize what you have understood and suggest a change in direction.*
- *Be honest about your time limitations.*
- *Acknowledge the value of what you have heard.*

These concerns about letting the genie out of the bottle are, we believe, more than offset by the clinical value of spending some time in pure listening. We have alluded to the healing power of listening for the patient and its positive impact on practitioner–patient relationships. Listening in this way can also do much to enrich your own practice. So rare are good listeners that even a little good-quality listening will open to you the rich inner experience of the people you serve. Few people are so privileged to share in the intimate inner world of so many fellow human beings. One such experience can uplift a day of otherwise routine practice. Good listening, you see, enriches not only the one to whom it is given as a gift but the giver as well.

LISTENING IN MI

Reflective listening itself—the pure listening skill—can be surprisingly effective in helping people change. If all that this book inspired you to do is to become a good listener in this skillful way, you would have an important gift to give to others. Once you are comfortable with reflective listening, *you can become more conscious and intentional about how you listen*, while retaining the warmth and genuine curiosity that lies at the heart of good listening. In MI, what you choose to reflect back to a patient can make a difference. The remainder of this chapter discusses what to reflect and why, when your goal is to encourage health behavior change.

In MI, what you choose to reflect back to a patient can make a difference.

Choosing What to Reflect

When you listen, even for a short time, you quickly discover that you have some decisions to make. As patients talk to you about their experience, they typically offer a rich array of material. You cannot begin to reflect all of it. Which comments will you pick, and how will you decide? Consider this exchange in which a practitioner opens the door with an invitation and then follows with pure listening.

PRACTITIONER [pediatric nurse or doctor]: Well, it looks like your boy's arm is going to be fine. I've patched up the wound and it should heal quickly. His tetanus vaccination is up to date, and the nurse is finishing up with him next door. Now, you mentioned that you've been more generally concerned about his behavior, and I have a few minutes before I see another patient. Tell me a little more about that.

PATIENT [mother]: It just seems that he's getting harder to control. He won't listen to us. Homework, meals, bedtime—it's all a struggle. He can't seem to sit still, and sometimes it seems like he just doesn't pay attention to what he's doing. That's how he cut his arm this time, you know. He wasn't looking where he was going and ran into our board fence with a rusty nail sticking out. I don't know how many times I've told my husband to fix that fence. [What part of all this might you choose to reflect at this point?]

PRACTITIONER: It's hard for you to manage him. [reflection]

PATIENT: Yes, and my husband and I don't agree on how to discipline him. He spanks him, and I think that's wrong. We've had a lot of fights lately.

PRACTITIONER: You and your husband. [reflection]

PATIENT: Yes. (*Tears come.*) I'm sorry, doctor. It's just all been so hard for me lately. I've heard about ADHD. One of the boys in his class has it, and I wonder if that might be what's wrong with him.

In the space of 1 minute of listening, the pediatrician suddenly has a rich array of issues from which to choose. Should she focus on the mother's feelings of distress, the struggles with homework and bedtime, the concerns about attention or activity level, the spanking, or perhaps the conflicts between husband and wife? How do you decide what to reflect?

For this particular situation, it could be useful to move from listening to agenda setting in the asking style, as described in Chapter 4. For present purposes, however, this conversation illustrates that a practitioner who listens must often choose what to reflect from among options. Within MI, there are some decision rules to help you in deciding what to reflect.

Reflect Resistance

When talking with a person who is ambivalent about change, you are bound to hear some resistance, some arguments for the status quo. The righting reflex is to refute these, to effectively argue against them and set the person straight. But as we've described earlier, if you argue for change, the patient will tend to voice the arguments against it. Because people who feel ambivalent have both sides of the argument within them, they will often back away from resistance when you reflect it nonjudgmentally. Even if they do not, you will get a clearer picture of the patients' reluctance. Here is a typical example from our work with problem drinkers:

PRACTITIONER: And tell me a little about your drinking. [open question]

PATIENT: Well, I do drink most days, but not that much, really.

PRACTITIONER: You're a pretty light drinker. [reflection]

PATIENT: Well, I'm not sure about that. I can hold it pretty well, more than most.

PRACTITIONER: You can drink a fair amount and it doesn't seem to affect you. [reflection]

PATIENT: Yeah, that's right. I can drink quite a bit.

PRACTITIONER: And you do sometimes. [reflection, continuing the paragraph]

PATIENT: Sure, I'll have five or six beers after work on the way home.

PRACTITIONER: [At this point the righting reflex is screaming, but the practitioner sticks with a guiding style to see what happens.] What do you think about drinking that much? [open question]

PATIENT: I don't really think about it that often.

PRACTITIONER: Sometimes you do, but not often. [reflection]

PATIENT: Well, sometimes I think, you know, I'm getting older and I ought to cut back.

PRACTITIONER: What have you noticed? [open question]

PATIENT: These stomach pains, like I've been having, and I guess I'm not as sharp sometimes in the mornings. But don't misunderstand, I don't have a *problem* with drinking.

PRACTITIONER: It hasn't really caused any problems for you. [reflection]

PATIENT: Well, I wouldn't say that. . . .

Patients who feel ambivalent have both sides of the argument within them, and they will often back away from resistance when you reflect.

The temptation is great to jump in using a directing style, and indeed it might not be entirely inappropriate for you to do so. Some clear information and advice from a health professional can make a difference. For example, you might well talk about safe drinking limits with this patient (see Chapter 6 on informing). We invite you, however, to try out this reflective way of responding to patient reluctance. Very often, it is then the patient who comes up with the other (pro-change) side of the argument, sometimes the very points you were about to voice yourself.

Reflect Change Talk

In the directing style, it is usually the practitioner who presents the case for change. Within a guiding style, it is the patient who does this. Change talk emerges, and this is what you reflect.

In Chapter 4 we discussed the strategic use of questions—asking those questions to which the answer is likely to be change talk. Such open questions often evoke a mixture of change talk and other language. Consider the forest meadow image we used earlier in this book. You are watching for the flowers, and as they appear, you pick some. In other words, what you particularly want to reflect, when you hear it, is change talk (statements of desire, ability, reasons, need, commitment, and taking steps). When you hear change talk, pick it out and reflect it back to the patient. In the following example, the patient's change talk is highlighted in ***boldface italic type***. Places where the practitioner uses reflective listening are indicated by ***[R]***.

PRACTITIONER: [audiologist]: Well, Mr. Sanchez, we're done with your testing, and there are some clear frequency ranges at which you're not hearing as well, which must be what your wife was noticing. That's not too unusual for your age, but the fact that there are these particular gaps suggests that there's something else going on besides normal aging. The nerve conductance test was normal, no apparent problem there. When have you been exposed to loud noises in your life, and how recently?

PATIENT: When I was younger I used to go trap shooting more, and we didn't always use the earplugs. Also I rode motorcycles—still do sometimes—and they can be loud.

PRACTITIONER: You've been around loud noises when shooting and riding motorcycles, which you still do sometimes. *[R]* What else?

PATIENT: I use some power tools, like a chain saw and a leaf blower. They're kind of loud.

PRACTITIONER: Right. And you don't always use ear protection. *[R]*

PATIENT: I never do, really, when I'm using tools.

PRACTITIONER: [resisting the temptation to immediately tell him why he should, and reflecting instead] It hasn't seemed important to you. *[R]*

PATIENT: I guess I haven't really thought about it. It's not all that loud, is it?

PRACTITIONER: [responding to the invitation to inform] I recommend that for anything above about 50 decibels people should protect their ears, and those tools would definitely be in that range. But it's kind of a hassle for you to put on ear protection every time you want to use a tool. *[R—still rolling with resistance rather than disagreeing with it]*

PATIENT: ***Well, not that big a deal, really. It's simple enough if it's important.***

PRACTITIONER: So popping in earplugs is something that you could do if you thought it was important enough. *[R]*

PATIENT: ***Sure. I could do that.*** [ability, not yet commitment]

PRACTITIONER: The problem has been that you didn't think it really matters that much. *[R]*

PATIENT: Or I just wasn't worrying about it, I guess. Didn't think about it.

PRACTITIONER: Well, while we are thinking about it together, let me ask you this. In what ways has your hearing loss been inconvenient for you so far? [This open question is particularly intended to evoke the patient's own motivations for behavior change.]

PATIENT: Not too much, really. ***My wife gets frustrated with me when I don't hear her.*** [reason]

PRACTITIONER: She gets a little irritated. ***[R]*** What else?

PATIENT: ***It's embarrassing sometimes when I don't understand what somebody said and I have to ask once or twice more. That seems to happen more often lately.*** [reason]

PRACTITIONER:Twice sometimes. ***[R]***

PATIENT: Especially if the person has like an accent or something, or if we're in a noisy restaurant. ***Sometimes I just pretend that I understand if I don't get it the second time, or don't ask at all, and then I miss things. I don't like that.*** [reason and desire]

PRACTITIONER: You told me that your wife thinks you may need a hearing aid, and perhaps you're wondering, too. ***[R]***

PATIENT: No, that would really be embarrassing. I don't want to go around with hardware in my ears.

PRACTITIONER: You don't like how hearing aids look. ***[R***—still rolling with resistance rather than arguing against it]

PATIENT: They make you look old, and also they're a hassle, the batteries and all that. And sometimes they squeak or screech out in public, and people look at you.

PRACTITIONER: Sounds like you hope you never have to wear one. ***[R]***

PATIENT: ***Well, probably sooner or later I'll need one,*** but I'd rather it be later. [need]

PRACTITIONER: So you might be interested in doings things now to protect the hearing you have left. ***[R]***

PATIENT: ***Yes, definitely.*** [beginning of commitment to behavior change]

PRACTITIONER: And it sounds like not wearing ear protection around noises—that wasn't because of embarrassment so much as just not thinking about it, not realizing that it's important. ***[R]***

PATIENT: ***Right. I can do that if it's going to keep me from needing a hearing aid.*** [ability]

PRACTITIONER: It would be worth it to you; seems like a small price to pay. ***[R]***

When you hear change talk, pick it out and reflect it back to the patient.

PATIENT: ***Sure, I'll do that.*** [commitment]

Working Through Ambivalence

Why take this time to reflect the patient's own motivations to change? The reason is that lifestyle patterns have substantial inertia, and the default is to continue unchanged. Past behavior predicts future behavior. We do not mean to be pessimistic about behavior change, because we see it all the time. It's just that unless something dislodges a current behavior pattern, it is likely to continue.

Isn't that an argument, then, for confronting patients with the consequences of their behavior, to jar them loose and rather forcefully persuade them to change? Although that sounds logical, such a frontal assault is actually more likely to entrench than to dislodge an established behavior, such as smoking, for example. When reflective listening is used within a guiding style, behavior change is more likely to occur.

Ambivalence can be a muddy meadow. People can stay mired there for some time. As discussed earlier, it's common to think about one reason why it might be good to make a change, then to think about a counterbalancing disadvantage of changing, and then to shut down and stop thinking about it. The guiding process of listening helps the person keep talking and moving in one direction toward change. You help the person keep thinking about and exploring the reasons (and desire, ability, need) for change instead of bouncing back and forth between pros and cons and then shutting down.

When listening is used within a guiding style, behavior change is more likely to occur.

How does that happen? When you reflect something that a person has said, you express interest in it and invite the person to say more about it, to elaborate. By being particularly interested in and focusing on the person's own motivations for behavior change—the flowers in the meadow—you encourage the person to keep on exploring and expanding on those.

You cannot know ahead of time what flowers will pop up, but bloom they do when you ask and listen. When you ask questions that elicit change talk, patients voice their own motivations for change and hear themselves expressing and exploring them. Then, when you reflect their own change talk, they hear you saying again (in slightly different words) what they themselves have said, and they explore it further. That lays the groundwork for yet one more use of listening to facilitate change.

Summaries: The Bouquet

Remember that in listening you periodically draw together what the person has said into a summary. In MI, these summaries have a particularly important function, because they contain the person's own motivations for change. You collect these flowers, the patients' own change talk statements, into a bouquet and periodically offer it back to them. It is particularly useful for the person to hear her or his own accumulated motivations for change collected all together, perhaps for the first time. This is different from the usual immobilizing process of ambivalence: thinking of one argument for change, then an argument against it, then stopping the process.

When listening, you periodically draw together what the person has said into a summary. In MI these summaries have a particularly important function, because they contain the person's own motivations for change.

All of this means that you need to be able to recognize a change talk flower when you see it (Chapter 3). Within MI, asking is used to elicit change talk (and eventually commitment), and listening is used to selectively reflect change talk and draw it into summaries. Here is an sample summary, following from the audiologist consultation earlier in this chapter:

PRACTITIONER: Let me see if I've heard you right, Mr. Sanchez. You've got some gaps in your hearing, and you've told me about past exposure to loud noises that might account for these. You notice that you are having more difficulty understanding people, especially if they speak with an accent or you're in a noisy place. Sometimes you have to ask people to repeat themselves once or twice, and you don't like that. This has also been a source of some friction between you and your wife, because she gets frustrated at having to repeat herself. She thinks maybe you should have a hearing aid, but you really don't want to do that yet because you would feel embarrassed, it might make you look older, and there are some practical hassles. You think you'll eventually need one, but you want to put it off as long as possible. So what you want to do is to preserve the hearing you have left as best you can, and for as long as you can, before it's time to get a hearing aid. So far so good?

PATIENT: That's right, yes. Well done! Nothing wrong with your hearing. (*Grins.*)

PRACTITIONER: So what makes sense to you is to take care of your hearing by using ear protection whenever you're going to be around loud noises. That would protect you from further damage and help keep these problems and embarrassments from getting worse. Is that what you're going to do?

PATIENT: Yes, I'll start using ear protection. [commitment]

PRACTITIONER: Great! Makes sense to me. Now how can I help you with that? Is there any information that would be useful about the kind of ear protection you can use, how to know when you should use it, anything like that? [asking permission to inform, a skill that we take up in the next chapter]

CONCLUSION

This chapter has described some of the breadth and depth of listening, with an emphasis on its use on the service of a guiding style. It's a practical skill that demands alertness, patience, and an ability to capture the patient's experience in a few well-chosen words. What you actually *do* is quite simple—you make a reflective listening statement—but your attention to detail and nuances of feeling will be appreciated by patients, and this allows them the freedom to resolve ambivalence about behavior change.

CHAPTER 6

Informing

Informing is probably the most commonly used tool in health care communication, woven into the fabric of most consultations. This chapter starts with some general considerations about informing and then turns to its use within MI.

SOME GENERAL CONSIDERATIONS

Informing is used in a wide range of situations. Here are some examples:

- Telling what has happened
- Explaining what is going to happen or what may happen
- Clarifying what something means
- Breaking bad news
- Sharing evidence
- Obtaining informed consent
- Mastering a task such as using a medical device
- Giving advice

"Some patients seem to hear, but others, I tell them time and again but it never seems to sink in." How difficult can it be to give patients information? Unfortunately, things do go wrong with this task. You may give what seem to be perfectly clear instructions, yet the patient does not fill a prescription or follow through with the next appointment. You go through what is or could be involved with a procedure, but later the patient is dissatisfied and complains that you did not adequately explain it. Many litigation cases in health care arise from disruptions of communication. And, commonly, the information you provide does not match the patient's hopes or expectations. "So you're not going to give me anything for this?" says the patient after your long explanation about managing her problem. "Aren't you going to do anything?"

A common-sense guideline is to be friendly and provide information in a clear and concise manner. Decades of research on information-giving and patient compliance have identified some essential ingredients of clarity when informing: Do not overload patients, provide simple information in chunks, be careful about using jargon and technical terms, check back to ensure that the patient has understood, and so on. Health care providers with little or no training in how to improve their informing skills often adhere to these guidelines but then find that things quickly become more complicated.

Things can and do go wrong with the informing process. You may give what seem to be perfectly clear instructions, yet the patient does not fill a prescription or follow through with the next appointment.

Put simply, patients may not be ready to hear what you have to say or may not agree with you about the importance of the information. They come from different cultures, backgrounds, and language groups, and a whole host of forces can affect their interest in and ability to absorb information you offer. These forces can include the following:

- *Bewilderment.* You provide information, and the patient just seems confused or bewildered. Is it the speed of the informing process, the patient's cognitive functioning, his or her attitude toward you, the words you used, or something else?
- *Passivity.* It seems to be going well until you take a more careful look at the patient, whose eyes are glazed over in a state of passivity, sitting back in the chair, waiting for you to get through your routine. Your duties sometimes demand that you get through large chunks of information with patients; for example, when you are required to inform patients for medical–legal and other good reasons. In the process of "getting through," you may yourself tune out a bit, feeling anxious, rushed, or bored. In the process it is easy to miss the cues that your patient has "switched off," that somewhere along the way you lost him or her. In the midst of informing, you may discover that your patient is no longer beside you.
- *High emotion.* Informing is easier when all is calm in the consultation and you have time to think and to do a good job. High emotion in yourself or your patient can change all that. Patients can feel angry,

frightened, or anxiously expectant. You may feel rushed, worried, tired, or irritated. High emotion blocks understanding.

• *Mood and distraction.* Relatedly, patients who are depressed may not hear and understand clearly what you are saying. Others may be distracted by recent events or worries and have trouble concentrating. (The same, of course, can happen to you.) The effects of alcohol, age, medication, or illicit drugs may impair the patient's ability to understand and remember.

Working Within a Relationship

Successful communication involves not just the transmission of technical expertise but interpersonal skills as well. A relationship, even if it lasts no more than a few minutes, lies at the heart of informing. The other two tools, asking and listening, are also needed to maintain working rapport with the patient, whose concerns, aspirations, and confusions express themselves in the consultation in many forms and affect your progress. "Information provision" is an inadequate description of what actually happens in practice. "Information exchange" is a more accurate phrase; you become immersed in improving your understanding, improving the patient's understanding, and reaching agreement about the issue at hand. This is a two-way process.

> *A relationship, even if it lasts no more than a few minutes, lies at the heart of informing.*

Here are a few practical guidelines for improving information exchange.

Slow Down, and Progress Can Be Quicker

The more hurried you feel, the less likely it is that you will be able to understand and respond to the challenges posed by patients. A common and understandable tendency is to hit "automatic pilot" and simply do the basics, giving patients the information that you feel it is your duty to provide. However, if you slow down a little and create the opportunity for both of you to be reflective, you will find the small silences very useful for giving the patient space and for giving yourself the time to make good judgments about the best way to get information across.

> *"Information provision" is an inadequate description of what actually happens in practice. "Information exchange" is a more accurate phrase.*

Better judgments can save time. Your questions and carefully chosen bits of information develop a quality of gravitas that patients pay attention to. One of us (Rollnick) attended an outpatient appointment with a worried spouse, in which the obstetrician conducted an examination and dealt with all of our concerns and questions in an *apparently* seamless consultation that lasted a matter of 10 minutes. It felt as though he had spent a much longer period of time with us. His manner was slow and thoughtful. A colleague once described this approach as being like a duck or swan gliding peacefully across the water, with legs nevertheless working hard under the surface. Skillful informing lay at the heart of the obstetrician's repertoire.

It's a Person, Not an Information Receptacle

This principle is so easily overlooked in the rushed world of everyday practice that it's worth the risk of stating the obvious. Well-intentioned efforts to "get through" and "make them understand" so that information "sinks in" often create the unfortunate impression of the patient as a passive recipient of information. The considerable skillfulness of practitioners who provide information closely tailored to the patient's personal needs often goes unappreciated.

Consider the Broader Priorities of the Patient

Inevitably, your concern is with your area of expertise, but the patient's priorities are much broader. He or she has to integrate the information and apply it to everyday life. What may be straightforward information to you can be much more for the patient. Simply conveying your acceptance of this reality can make a substantial difference to the outcome. How does the information that you are providing fit in with the patient's life and perspective?

Positive Messages Matter

Often in health care information can be divided into good news and not-so-good news. For example, when you are informing a patient of a new diagnosis, there will likely be a mix of troubling information with some positive messages. How do you strike the balance between the two? Some practitioners are concerned that providing positive messages might "gloss over the hard facts" and compromise frankness. Including truthful positive messages, however, can actually increase a patient's receptiveness to hard facts. Consider the difference between:

"If you continue to smoke, breathing is only going to become more difficult."

and

"If you stop smoking, you may find that breathing is easier."

Consider the Amount of Information

People vary widely in their desire for information. When facing a surgical procedure, some patients want great detail about what will be done. They want to know exactly what to expect, and having more information decreases their distress. Some practices maintain a video library showing common procedures and lend these to patients who want this level of detail. Other patients prefer to know as little detail as possible, and having more information frightens them. It makes sense, then, to ask patients their preferences about being informed. On a particular topic, how much do they already know? What would they like to know, and in what detail? Whether to withhold or provide information is not a decision to make by yourself. Find out your patient's wishes.

Deliver Information with Care

Give the message in an accessible way. If the medium of the instruction is the spoken word, make sure the words are understandable to the patient. Avoid the abbreviations much loved by health care practitioners. Avoid technical terms when possible, and, when not possible, check as to whether your patient knows their meaning. Avoid words your patient may consider "infantile." If you use written material, it should be appropriate to the patients' educational level, vision, time, and anxiety state.

Sometimes verbal instruction is best; sometimes a combination of media will be best. A leaflet, a website, and a book, for example, may complement an initial verbal instruction. Some patients may value the opportunity to tape-record your instructions. Check with the patient about what medium or combination of media best suits him or her.

Always use informing in combination with asking and listening. Check: Are the messages being received by your patients? Have they heard you? Have they understood what you are trying to convey? How is the pace of information delivery suiting your patients? A simple question such as "How are we doing so far?" will often help you to decide how best to proceed.

Directing with Care

A directing style can be used in routine practice to exchange information to very good effect. This involves more than just being pleasant and clear, and the countless examples of good practice observable in busy consulting rooms bear witness to this fact. It involves attentiveness and skillful responding to both your mood and needs and those of the patient.

Skillful informing is more than just being pleasant and clear. It involves attentiveness and skillful responding to both your mood and needs and those of the patient.

INFORMING WITHIN MI

MI is based on a guiding style, and a competent guide provides good information but does it in a particular way. This section offers some specific guidelines on how to inform within MI.

Ask Permission

Providing information *with permission* from the patient is fundamental to the use of a guiding style. Informing is most likely to go wrong and elicit resistance when the patient is unready or unwilling to receive it. Within the principle of respecting patient autonomy (Chapter 2), the practitioner informs or advises only when he or she has permission to do so. There are three ways to obtain such permission.

The first and simplest form of permission involves your patient *asking* you for information or advice. Here the patient has opened the door for you. Sometimes we are still a bit cautious under this circumstance and first ask what the patient already knows (information) or what ideas the patient may have for how to proceed (advice). In general, though, it is fine to inform when the patient asks you to do so.

A second way is to ask for permission to inform. This is analogous to knocking on the door before you enter. Before you charge into informing or advising, ask if that would be all right with the patient.

> "Would you like to know some things that other patients have done?"
>
> "Would it be all right if I tell you one concern I have about this plan?"
>
> "There are several things that you can do to keep the level of sugar in your blood under control. Do you want to hear them, or are there other things that we should talk about first?"
>
> "May I make a suggestion?"

Asking for permission in this way has several good effects. First, it directly honors and reinforces patients' autonomy and active involvement in their own health care. It emphasizes the collaborative nature of your relationship. It also lowers resistance. Asking permission to offer information or advice often makes the patient more willing to hear it. Furthermore, it can give you important information. If there is something much more pressing on the patient's mind, you're likely to find out about it.

> *Asking for permission has several good effects. It directly honors and reinforces patients' autonomy and active involvement in their own health care. It emphasizes the collaborative nature of your relationship. It also lowers resistance.*

In most situations, these first two ways of getting permission will suffice. That leaves the less common situation in which you feel impelled to give information and advice and are not be willing to accept a "no" answer when you ask for permission. There are several things you can do in this case:

- *Announcing.* One good option is simply to tell the truth. "There is something that I need to tell you here."
- *First choice.* Another possibility is to ask the patient whether you should do this now or whether there is something else that he or she wants to talk about *first.* This implies that sooner or later you are going to do the informing or advising, but it still gives the patient some latitude about when it happens.
- *Prefacing.* Another good option is to preface the informing or advising with a comment that directly acknowledges the patient's autonomy. Telling them that they are free to disregard what you are about to say somehow makes them more willing to hear it.

> "I don't know if this will make sense to you or not . . .
> "This may or may not concern you, but . . . "
> "You can tell me what you think of this idea . . . "

Obviously these three components can be used in combination:

> "I have a concern about your plan that you may or may not share, but I feel like I need to express it. Would it be all right if I explained it now, or is there something else that you want to ask about first?"

Obtaining the patient's permission in one of these three ways is a fundamental element when informing within MI.

Offer Choices

When informing, offer choices when possible. This supports patient autonomy. For example, a rock-climbing guide, committed to helping people learn by making their own judgments, might say: "If you look above you to the left, you will see that pointed rock, which could be unstable. One option is to reach up and try it. Another is to move over to your right, where you can stretch across to that ledge. Which move makes more sense to you?" Expert information is used to help the person make an informed choice. That's what we mean by informing in the service of guiding. You stop short of telling someone what to do; instead, you provide useful, well-tailored choices.

> "It's a common fear that exercise might actually cause another heart attack. If you do this gently, there's no evidence at all that this is harmful. It's a question of what will suit you. Some of our patients walk longer distances each day, some use a machine at home, others come down here to use our machines. It's your choice. I wonder what would make sense to you right now, or is this all a bit too much too soon?"

This illustrates a broader guideline about offering choices within MI. When you discuss options, offer several simultaneously. There is an obvious trap in discussing choices one at a time. You present one possibility, and the patient tells you what is wrong with it. So then you raise another option, and the patient tells you why that one won't work. Suddenly you are back in the persuasion trap in which you argue for change and the patient argues against it. Instead, offer a variety of options, and ask the person to choose among them. "Pick a card, any card" creates a different mindset from, "What do you think about this possibility?"

When you discuss options, offer several simultaneously.

Talk about What Others Do

When giving information, particularly if it contains implications for action, consider the value of talking about how this has affected *other* patients, and avoid suggesting what the patient should do. This is an example of avoiding the righting reflex. Patients then have the freedom to say what might work for them, usually in the form of change talk. This leaves you in a position of neutrality. In other words, you provide, and the patient interprets. For example, there's a difference between:

Avoid the righting reflex by talking about how the information has affected other patients, and avoid suggesting what the patient should do. This leaves you in a position of neutrality. In other words, you provide, and the patient interprets.

"You clearly need to cut down on your intake of fatty foods, and stopping smoking is a top priority as well."

and

"Some patients in your situation reduce their intake of fatty foods, others tackle their smoking. I wonder what makes sense to you? . . . "

Two Strategies for Informing

Chunk–Check–Chunk

A common exhortation in the teaching of students in health care is to use the "chunk–check–chunk" approach to providing information to patients. You provide a chunk of information, check patient understanding, provide another chunk, and so on. Its value lies in respectful checking to see that the patient has understood before moving on to the next chunk of information. It is used most often in the service of a directing style, in which the "check" phase is used merely to ensure that the patient has understood the information, which is appropriate in many circumstances. When it comes to behavior change and the use of a guiding style, the "check" step involves a bit more than asking, "Got it?" Rather, you stop to ask for the patient's perspective. What does the patient think about this chunk? Is there any part of it that the patient did not understand or would like to ask about further?

The chunk–check–chunk approach is most commonly used in the service of a directing style, quite appropriately in many circumstances. However, it can be adapted for use in the service of a guiding style to talk about behavior change.

PRACTITIONER: So it does look like you have some nerve damage in your feet, and there are some things you might want to do to protect your feet. I recommend that you not walk around barefoot, but wear slippers, even at home. Be careful about hot water. Use padded socks, and examine your feet once a day to look for any cuts, blisters, or other injuries. Use a mirror if you need to in order to see the soles of your feet. [chunk] That's quite a few recommendations from me! Do they make sense to you? [check]

PATIENT: Yes, I think so.

PRACTITIONER: Is there anything in this you want to ask me about? [checking further]

PATIENT: Well, you said to be careful about hot water. Do you mean that I shouldn't take a warm bath? Is hot water somehow bad for my feet?

PRACTITIONER: Thanks for asking. No, it's not that warm water is bad for you. The danger is that sometimes people use their feet to test the temperature of water in a bath. That can be a problem. I see patients with diabetes who have burned their feet badly before realizing that the water was too hot. The feet become insensitive, and people get burned before they realize it. [chunk] Does that make sense? [check]

PATIENT: Oh, I see. It's just to make sure I don't burn my feet without realizing it. OK, I'll be careful. I guess I'll use my hand or something.

PRACTITIONER: Good! Now if you happen to find any cut, blister, or other wound on your feet, or if you have any other concerns about your feet, please come in to see me right away. [chunk] Will you do that? [check]

PATIENT: Yes. I don't want to have problems with my feet, so I need to check them daily and let you know if I see anything.

PRACTITIONER: Right. Very good. And are you OK with the padded socks idea? [check]

This rhythm of asking for patients' responses in between chunks is good for several reasons. First, it continues to actively engage patients in their own care, even when you are informing. It communicates patience and respect. It also helps you detect and correct misunderstandings that you might otherwise miss. Too often the information-giving process in health care goes primarily in one direction, from the practitioner to the patient. The patient is rendered a passive recipient, which makes it easy to overlook miscommunication and inhibits the exploration and expression of motivation to change. Chunk–check–chunk can turn the informing process into a conversation rather than a lecture, at least when "check" means a genuine checking in for the patient's understanding and perspectives.

Elicit–Provide–Elicit

This phrase provides a different guideline for information exchange that is more congruent with the principles of MI. It places considerable value on drawing from the patients what they need and want to know and, critically, what new information means to them. This again emphasizes patients' active involvement in their own health care and is intended to enhance motivation for behavior change. Elicit–provide–elicit (EPE) is not meant to be a linear sequence of steps but rather a cyclical process of guiding through information exchange. Although it revolves around informing, EPE also requires both asking (often open questions) and listening.

In EPE, the information exchange begins with you asking patients an open question to focus your informing. We suggest two general forms of this eliciting question. The first is to ask, "What would you most like to know about ______?" Here you invite the patient to tell you what seems most important to know from his or her own perspective. A second form is to ask, "What do you already know about ______?" This latter form has several advantages. It can save you time and prevent you from lecturing patients about what they already know. It allows you to correct misconceptions that you might otherwise overlook. Furthermore, having the patient voice this knowledge often serves as a form of change talk by at least implicitly stating the need for health behavior change and the consequences of not doing so.

The second part of the EPE cycle—provide—involves providing information in a manageable chunk. If you have asked what the patient would like to know, you already have permission to inform. The second opening question—what the patient already knows—also often leads to a request for you to inform, but if there's any doubt you can simply ask permission: "Would you like for me to tell you a bit about . . . ?" *Focus initially on information more than your own interpretation of what it means for this patient.* You may talk about other patients' experience as part of this information-providing step.

Focus initially on information more than your own interpretation of what it means for this patient. You may talk about other patients' experience as part of this information-providing step.

The third part of EPE is again to ask an open question to elicit the patient's response to the chunk of information you just provided. Some possibilities are:

"What do you make of that?"
"What does this mean for you?"
"What more would you like to know?"

The difference between using a directing style and the elicit–provide–elicit framework is in your attitude. Often in chunk–check–chunk, the mindset is that there is a certain amount of information that you, the expert, want to provide to the patient. The "check" questions are mostly to make sure that the patient is getting what you say. You give the information, and the patient's job is to understand it.

EPE involves a more collaborative mindset that is appropriate when the topic is health behavior change. The question in your mind is not so much how to get information across as how to help the patient make sense of it and make good decisions about behavior and stick to them. To do this, you find out about the patient's own concerns, current knowledge base, and interests in knowing more. One way of striking this balance is to remember the following: You have considerable expertise in what has been good for other patients in similar circumstances; your patients, on the other hand, are usually more expert about what works best for them. Keeping this in mind can be very helpful. Fill in the information gaps and see what the patient makes of it all.

You have considerable expertise in what has been good for other patients in similar circumstances; your patients, on the other hand, are usually more expert about what works best for them.

One of the very first applications of MI involved using exactly this EPE approach. We advertised the availability of a "free checkup for drinkers who wonder whether alcohol is harming them in any way." The announcement made it clear that this was not a treatment program and that the person was free to decide what, if anything, to do about the personal health information provided. A surprising number of people responded, seeking this "drinker's checkup," which included a variety of measures of physiological and psychological functions that tend to be affected earlier by heavy drinking. A counselor then met just once with the patient to present the findings of the checkup, comparing the person's own scores with normal ranges. Instead of giving advice and concluding what the patient should do, the counselor asked for the person's own interpretation of the findings, filling in any further information requested. Virtually all of those who responded were heavy drinkers and were already experiencing harmful consequences. In randomized trials, patients who received the drinker's checkup showed significant reductions in drinking without further intervention relative to those assigned to a waiting list for the checkup. It also mattered how the counselor presented the feedback. Within an empathic EPE style, patients voiced about twice as much change talk and half as much resistance relative to a more directing and confronting style. In fact, the more the counselor confronted, the more the client was drinking at follow-up.

You provide and the patient interprets.

One useful guideline is to consider the difference between a "teachable moment" and a "learning opportunity." The former is often driven by an insertion approach to information giving, whereas the latter characterizes many of the qualities embedded in the EPE framework.

Beware the Righting Reflex

Again, it is wise to tame your righting reflex when informing. Some practitioners believe that if someone is sufficiently scared, he might change or take greater notice of the information provided. However, fear is a complex motivation, and scare tactics can backfire. A common response to fear is to become defensive and shut down, as illustrated by some patients whose response to bad news about their health is to have a drink or light up a cigarette at the first opportunity. One patient we interviewed told us, "Every time I go in there, he tells me that smoking is bad for me, as if he's telling me some new breathtaking secret, yet I see the health warning on the packet every time I light up." There is very little evidence for the belief that people will change if you can just make them feel bad (scared, ashamed, humiliated) enough. To the contrary, it is the supportive, compassionate, empathic practitioner who is most effective in inspiring behavior change.

Another pitfall of the righting reflex is premature focus. It can put the patient off when you rush in with your perspective or solution: "You've got to take a proton pump inhibitor to really get on top of your gastric reflux." Some problems may not be major problems from the viewpoint of a practitioner, but they are for a patient, and vice versa. In many situations, the best solutions come from the patients, not from practitioners rushing in to solve the problem: "Well, actually, I don't like taking medicine, and I've already started losing weight, and my reflux is already much improved, thank you!"

There is very little evidence for the belief that people will change if you can just make them feel bad (scared, ashamed, humiliated) enough. To the contrary, it is the supportive, compassionate, empathic practitioner who is most effective in inspiring behavior change.

PRACTICAL EXAMPLES

Here are a few examples from everyday practice. The chunk–check–chunk approach is used in the service of a directing style, to highlight its vulnerability to the righting reflex when talking about behavior change, and to provide a strong contrast with the EPE approach.

Promoting Adherence

Research on medication adherence has pinpointed the importance of clear communication about medicine use and the need to consider the patient's concerns. This is particularly challenging when you are pressed for time, knowing that you have little control over forces outside the consultation that influence adherence, such as cultural values, social conditions, personal habits, memory, and so on. The EPE framework is intended to enhance your ability to absorb and respond constructively to these challenges. The hypothesis is that adherence will be improved, because a guiding style and the use of this framework elicit the patient's own motivations to address these problems.

Here is an example that illustrates the contrast between the chunk–check–chunk approach used in the service of a directing style and the EPE strategy used in the service of a guiding style.

Chunk–Check–Chunk

Practitioner: Nurse, counselor, doctor, pharmacist, or patient advocate.
Setting: Treatment for HIV/AIDS.

PRACTITIONER: It's very important for your health that you take the medicines properly. [chunk] Have you been taking them properly? [check; closed question]

PATIENT: Yes, well, it's difficult to take everything at the right time, and I am starting to feel a bit better, so that's good.

PRACTITIONER: You know that you need to take them every day, at exactly the right time, and you must not miss any, even if you are feeling better [chunk]. How often are you taking the medicines? [check; closed question]

PATIENT: Yes, but it's hard, you see. If my mother sees me taking them, then she will figure out what's going on, and that will bring bad things for me. She doesn't know, you see.

PRACTITIONER: Maybe you could go into the bathroom to take them. [chunk]

PATIENT: Yes, but I also have the baby, and it gets very busy to do everything just at the right time.

PRACTITIONER: How often have you been missing your medications? [check; closed question]

Comment: The righting reflex has its limitations, despite the well-intentioned efforts of a concerned practitioner. Indeed, the more concerned you feel, the easier it is to fall into this trap. With a shift in style, the chunk–check–chunk approach could be adapted constructively for use in this kind of consultation. In this next example, we illustrate the use of the EPE strategy.

Elicit–Provide–Elicit

Practicer and setting: Same as above.

PRACTITIONER: How are you feeling about the medicines you are taking? [elicit; open question]

PATIENT: I take them like you told me to.

PRACTITIONER: Many people in your situation find it hard to take them all at the right time. [provide; what others do] What's the best way for you to take them? How do you do it? [elicit; open question]

PATIENT: I try to take them like you said, but it's not so easy, with my mother around all the time. She doesn't know, you see.

PRACTITIONER: It must be hard for you to keep this secret and take your medicine at the right time. [listening]

PATIENT: That's right. I can't tell her now. Is it a big problem if I miss some of the tablets?

PRACTITIONER: Actually, that is a problem. For these medicines to work, people have to keep taking them faithfully, and it's important to take them right on time. [provide after permission-granting question from the patient] Does that make sense to you? [elicit; open question]

PATIENT: So you say that even if I feel better I should take the medicines all the time?

PRACTITIONER: That's right, it's very important to take them faithfully even if you start to feel better. [provide] What's going to be the best way for you to do that? [elicit; open question]

PATIENT: It's my mother always looking at me, and if I tell her I've got HIV it will be bad. She might even kick me out, or try to take away my baby.

PRACTITIONER: You don't feel ready to tell her about this. [listening; reflecting resistance]

PATIENT: No, not now. Maybe later, but I don't feel strong enough.

PRACTITIONER: I wonder how you can manage, then, to take your medications as you need to? [elicit change talk]

PATIENT: One thing I do is go in my bedroom and close the door when it's time for my medicine. [change talk]

PRACTITIONER: That sounds like a possibility. Can I tell you what some mothers do? [asking permission to provide; talk about what others do]

Comment: The second example did indeed take a little longer, perhaps a minute more. However, this does not need to become a protracted counseling process. Most patients understand that you are busy. After a few minutes of eliciting and providing, you can usually summarize what they have said and shift to another topic or issue. In this case, it might have to be the difficult matter of disclosure of HIV status.

Sharing Test Results

Another example of using the EPE framework is in informing patients about test results. Opportunities for discussing test results exist across the board in both acute care and long-term-condition management. These often have implications for medicine use, adherence, and health behavior change. In Chapter 2 we described the case of Stefan, a 14-year-old boy who attends the diabetes clinic to receive the news of his blood test result from a practitioner who feels strongly, and with genuine concern, that this information could have a bearing on his future well-being and health. A chunk–check–chunk approach used in the service of a directing style often restricts attention only to that which is of interest to the practitioner. The patient usually senses this and responds accordingly. Stefan's experience of the contrasting approaches is illustrated here.

Chunk–Check–Chunk

Practitioner: Doctor or nurse.
Setting: Treatment for diabetes.
Challenge: The practitioner feels strongly that the test result has important implications for health.

PRACTITIONER: [after some preliminary friendly everyday conversation] Now, Stefan, I'd like to move on to the blood test results, if I may, which have just come in from the lab. I know we have been through this before, but it's important to keep an eye on these to see how you're doing. [chunk] Is that OK with you? [check]

PATIENT: Yes, OK.

PRACTITIONER: Well it's 11.5 today, so that's a rise from last time I saw you. Let me see, that was 3 months ago, and then it was 9.2, so that's quite a big increase. [chunk] Do you understand? [check]

PATIENT: Yeah.

PRACTITIONER: Now we need to talk about what we can do about this, because we don't want to see you back here in the hospital when you're older with all sorts of problems. I mean, it's not that I don't like seeing you (*laughs*), but you know what I mean, this result tells us that all is not well with your diabetes. [chunk] Do you see what I mean? [check]

PATIENT: Yeah, well, you know, I do try, like, I do take my injections like you tell me.

PRACTITIONER: What's most important is that you really get on top of monitoring your sugars and giving yourself the insulin exactly like we agreed, four times a day. Last time we agreed we would go for tight control because this will give you the best chance of avoiding problems later on, with your eyes and other organs. [chunk]

PATIENT: Yes, I see, I do try my best.

PRACTITIONER: Well, it's a bit of a problem. This test result is up from the last time I saw you. [chunk] Do you understand what that means? [check]

PATIENT: Yea, sometimes that happens, I guess, but I am trying.

Comment: In this example, a clearly concerned practitioner, pressed for time, sacrificed a few minutes of listening and rapport building at the outset (a following style) for the immediate use of an installation approach to informing. The righting reflex prevailed, however, and the patient closed right down in the face of a meeting that felt a bit like a visit to the school principal's office. Chunk–check–chunk can be used to greater effect with more listening in the "check" phase. The EPE sequence is often more rewarding.

Elicit–Provide–Elicit

Practitioner and setting: Same as above.

PRACTITIONER: [after some preliminary following of the patient's account of his everyday life] I'd like to talk about the blood test result, but we can first talk about any aspect of your life and diabetes. School, home, how are things going? [brief agenda setting]

PATIENT: OK. I get by, but I get embarrassed at school, like if I have to ask the soccer coach to leave to go get something to eat.

PRACTITIONER: I remember you like your soccer. So this is embarrassing for you. [listening]

PATIENT: It's OK, most of my friends understand, but the coach, he makes a thing of it.

PRACTITIONER: He makes you feel abnormal and stand out. [listening]

PATIENT: Yeah. So I try to keep going without doing anything about it.

PRACTITIONER: And that's not always easy. [listening]

PATIENT: Most of the time it's OK, but sometimes I just have to stop, and he makes a big deal of it and embarrasses me.

PRACTITIONER: Would it be helpful for me to have a talk with this teacher, or would you prefer to handle this on your own?

PATIENT: No, I'll handle it.

PRACTITIONER: Well, then, what would you like to know about the blood results? [elicit]

PATIENT: Not much, because I knew it was going to be high today.

PRACTITIONER: You were a little nervous about this one. [listening]

PATIENT: Yeah. (*Laughs nervously.*)

PRACTITIONER: What would you guess the number is, if it was 9.2 last time?

PATIENT: 10?

PRACTITIONER: A little higher!

PATIENT: That bad?

PRACTITIONER: 11.5. It's quite a bit higher than usual. You had been doing quite well in trying for tight control. A useful idea for some young people is to think of just a few small things that are manageable in helping them achieve tighter control. [provide]

PATIENT: Oh.

PRACTITIONER: You're not too shocked about this. What sense do you make of it? [elicit]

PATIENT: I haven't been eating right, and I haven't been monitoring my sugars very often. I hate doing it, I hate going off to the toilet in school to do the monitoring.

PRACTITIONER: You try to cope with the diabetes, and you want to feel normal. [listening]

PATIENT: Yeah, I know, its hard, I'm not doing very well, and my eating is not right.

PRACTITIONER: You know that you haven't been taking good enough care of yourself. [listening] How can I help? [elicit]

PATIENT: What do you think . . . ?

Comment: With the patient's concerns center stage, the practitioner now has an opportunity to guide him to find ways of managing without standing out among his peers. There may not be easy solutions here, but the service being offered to the boy is at least attuned to his needs. Information provision was a central part of that process.

What Does This Information Mean *for Me*?

Sometimes patients feel sufficiently provided with information itself but are less clear about its personal implications. This is where your ability to elicit their own thinking about the information is critical, and this can be done in just a minute or two. The guideline to follow is this: You provide the information, and you encourage the patient to interpret it:

Practitioner: Doctor or nurse
Setting: Primary care, a cholesterol result
Challenge: Simple solutions in the mind of the practitioner appear more difficult for the patient. How do you elicit decisions about behavior change in a brief consultation?

PRACTITIONER: Well, Mr. Brazier, the cholesterol test is back, and it is still slightly raised. Just so I don't concentrate on the wrong stuff, I wonder if I could ask you what you already know about raised cholesterol and what you would like to know? Are you happy to discuss this now? [elicit] Or would it be better if I gave you something to read in the meanwhile and we discussed things, perhaps together with your wife, next time?

PATIENT: No, I'm fine to talk now. Actually I know a quite a bit about cholesterol already. My brother, as it turns out, had a test, and his cholesterol was raised a bit, so we looked on the Internet together.

PRACTITIONER: You understand about the problems with high cholesterol. So what do you think this test result means for you? [elicit]

PATIENT: Well, I'm not really sure what's best to do about it.

PRACTITIONER: What is confusing you about this? [elicit]

PATIENT: OK, it's raised, but how do I get it down, without stopping smoking or changing my diet, or have I got this wrong?

PRACTITIONER: No, you've got it right, those kinds of changes can make a big difference. [provide]

PATIENT: But I am worried about what effect quitting smoking may have on my diet.

PRACTITIONER: So you are worried that quitting smoking might increase your weight and be bad for you [listening].

PATIENT: Yes, that's it. My weight shot up when I quit last year. Is it better to quit smoking even if I pick up a bit of weight, or should I just focus on my eating for now and leave the smoking for later?

PRACTITIONER: Well, on average, the biggest risk by far for most people of having a stroke or heart attack, especially when they have raised cholesterol, is smoking. Smokers who have raised cholesterol, even if they are eating well, have a greatly increased risk of having a heart attack or stroke. [provide] So what do you make of this? [elicit]

PATIENT: Well, I guess I kind of knew that while diet is important, overall, smoking is probably worse than the eating, and even if I gain some, if I crack the smoking, overall, I will be better off. To be honest, I have been worried about my smoking for a while now. My dad died of a heart attack. OK, he was old, but now with my brother also having raised cholesterol and now me. . . .

PRACTITIONER: I can tell you how other patients like you have stopped smoking, and what might help. Would that be of interest?

PATIENT: OK, I guess so.

Comment: By going back and forth between eliciting and providing, the practitioner moves the discussion along toward behavior change while taking into account the patient's concerns.

Messages of Hope in 60 Seconds*

In the course of everyday practice, there is often much to discuss with a patient, and you do not want to completely neglect the topic of behavior change. In Chapter 1 we mentioned four core principles of MI, the last of which is to support optimism and hope for change. Even when a pa-

---

* We thank Drs. Gary Rose and Chris Dunn for helping us construct this dialogue.

tient is not ready to change, simply talking about what he or she could do to make a difference can help. You are planting a seed of hope.

Practitioner: Doctor or nurse.
Setting: Primary care.
Challenge: Depression and lifestyle change: A man who lives alone and works in a job he describes as unbearable presents in primary care with low mood. He agrees to medication and returns for a follow-up appointment. You discuss his situation, and because he is also obese, you decide to provide advice in 60 seconds about lifestyle change while still using a guiding style.

PRACTITIONER: You were talking about feeling low in energy, and I am wondering if I could briefly ask you about your diet and exercise. [elicit]

PATIENT: OK.

PRACTITIONER: Little changes, little new habits in either of these things will help with mood, and they would also help reduce your weight, which is a concern for me. [provide] These things are all linked, if you see what I mean.

PATIENT: Yes, I do see.

PRACTITIONER: This is really your choice, and I hope you don't mind my raising it. I'm wondering, how do you really feel about this? [elicit]

PATIENT: I know what you are saying, but I don't know, really, it's all I can do to get out of bed on time and make it through the day.

PRACTITIONER: It takes a lot of your energy just to get through the day. In fact, you don't feel like you have lots of choices. [listening]

PATIENT: Yeah, I mean the effort to do all these things. . . . I can't see myself changing. . . .

PRACTITIONER: You wish you had more energy, but you don't. [listening]

PATIENT: That's exactly right.

PRACTITIONER: There might well be some things you could do to feel better and have more energy, but you will know when the right time is to try them. You've agreed to come back and see me, and for now, you're not sure how to make changes in diet and exercise. I don't want you to feel guilty about not making any changes. We've got time, and perhaps you can just think about what small changes might make sense to you. We can talk more about this next time, and I'll do whatever I can to help you get through this difficult time.

PATIENT: Thank you very much.

Comment: If you were to take a few more minutes, you could evoke and explore further some of the patient's own motivations to improve diet and exercise, but even planting the seed is helpful.

WITHIN YOUR GRASP

A great deal of modern health care focuses on providing patients with information, and it often does so in a way that fails to evoke behavior change. The search is on for new media aids and technologies to convey information to patients more effectively and efficiently. Meanwhile, an answer may be right there within your grasp—to mix skillful informing with listening and asking for the patient's own perspectives. You have the potential to shift style from directing to guiding when appropriate. This requires a shift away from feeling responsible for the patients' changing behavior and toward helping them realize (and verbalize) their own reasons and means for change. The prescription that "You have to make these changes" is an empty one, for, in fact, patients do not have to do what they are told. They make choices. Informing from your expertise is still an important part of MI, from which you help patients ask themselves, "What does this information mean for me? What changes should I and can I make?" Seen in this light, informing can be a powerful tool indeed. The more active the patient is in this discussion, the better.

CONCLUSION

This chapter has described the rationale for using information close to the heart of good practice in MI. The elicit–provide–elicit framework has been presented as one way of conducting the discussion so that the patient is an active participant in making decisions about behavior change. In Part III we turn to the integration of these skills in motivational interviewing (Chapters 7–9) and conclude with attention to how the method might fit into the broader service you deliver to patients (Chapter 10).

PART III

PUTTING IT ALL TOGETHER

CHAPTER 7

Integrating the Skills

We have discussed how communication skills that you commonly use in ordinary practice—asking, listening, and informing—can be applied to guiding patients toward behavior change. We have also discussed how the righting reflex and the directing style, appropriate in so many situations, can backfire when you would like a patient to consider behavior change. A switch to a guiding style allows you to explore the patient's *own* motivations for health behavior change and encourages the patient to voice them to you. This need not take a long time; it is just a different and often more effective method of communicating when the challenge is to encourage behavior change.

Within MI, a specialized use of the guiding style, you set an agenda and then *ask* about particular things (Chapter 4), namely, the patient's own desire, ability, reasons, and need (DARN) to make a change, such as stopping smoking. Instead of asking patients why they have not stopped smoking, you are interested in why they might want to, how they would do it, what their reasons would be, and how important it is to them.

In MI, ask about the patients' own desire, ability, reasons, and need (DARN); ask why they might want to change, how they would do it, what their reasons are, and how important it is to them.

Each such question is followed by *listening*, by reflecting back in somewhat different words what the person has told you and perhaps anticipating what may lie beneath the surface of what you have heard ("continuing the paragraph"; see Chapter 5). You are listening in particular for the "flowers," the patient's own DARN statements. Each time you hear one, you tuck it away in memory, and then you offer them back to the person in a "bouquet" summary (Chapter 5). You will also still be using informing but probably less than is accustomed practice. In the style of a guide, informing is done with permission and by helping the patient to express what the information means for him or her (Chapter 6).

CREATIVE COMBINATIONS

No one works purely with one communication skill. Consultation involves moving back and forth flexibly among asking, listening, and informing. Consider the following combinations of the three core skills. The aim here is not to suggest that these combinations are guidelines for structuring the consultation; rather, it is simply to encourage you to recognize different patterns of skills usage.

Informing and Asking

Practitioner: Nurse, doctor, counselor.
Setting: Trauma.
Challenge: To encourage the patient, a young woman, to consider the role played by alcohol in a car accident.

PRACTITIONER: [at the bedside of a young woman] We've got you stabilized now, Heather, but you're going to be in this specialized unit for a day or two, and then probably in the hospital for a few more days after that until it's safe for you to go home. [informing] So tell me what happened that led to the crash? [asking]

PATIENT: I don't remember the accident itself. I just woke up here in this bed with my legs up like this. I remember getting into the car, though. We were at a party, out meeting guys, and by the time we headed home it was after midnight. I hadn't had too much to drink, just two or three beers all night, but I know Lisa had a lot more. I should have been the one driving (*crying*).

PRACTITIONER: You were both badly hurt, but your injuries are worse. We sent Lisa home, and she's going to be all right. You have some internal injuries, though, and your legs are both broken in several places, so you'll be on crutches for a couple of months at least after we get you home. [informing] Is there anything I can do for you? How is your pain? [asking]

PATIENT: I'm all right—I feel pretty drugged up. Just get me out of here.

PRACTITIONER: We'll get you home as soon as we can. I see this a lot, you know—people riding with someone who shouldn't be driving. [informing]

PATIENT: Yeah. Lisa shouldn't have been driving.

PRACTITIONER: Did you realize that at the time, when you got in the car with her? [asking]

PATIENT: I kind of knew. She drank a lot more than I did.

PRACTITIONER: I'm worried about you. Not just because of your injuries. They could have been a lot worse. But of all the people who come in here, how many would you guess are back within a year, injured again? [asking, implicit permission to inform]

PATIENT: I don't know. Not very many, I would think.

PRACTITIONER: About one out of four we see here again in this trauma center within 1 year. [informing]

PATIENT: Wow! Really! Why?

PRACTITIONER: People who drink and drive also tend to take other risks, but the biggest risk is that they get in another crash. And it's not just the drinking drivers. Like you, those who ride with drinking drivers, even if they were sober themselves, wind up back here at the same rate as the drivers. [informing] What sense do you make of that? [asking]

PATIENT: I can see it, really. It could just as well have been me. I've been drinking plenty of nights before driving home.

Asking and Listening

This conversation with Heather continues, with the trauma surgeon now intermixing asking and listening. Remember that listening, as discussed in Chapter 5, is not a passive process but one in which the listener actively reflects back what the person has said. Notice also that this reflecting process is not limited to what the patient has actually said; good listening statements may continue the paragraph or make a guess about unspoken meaning.

PRACTITIONER: Tell me a little more about that. [asking; open question]

PATIENT: Well, last night—it was last night, wasn't it?—I just didn't feel like drinking much, so I only had a few brews.

PRACTITIONER: Just two or three beers, because you weren't feeling well. [listening, and a guess]

PATIENT: I didn't feel bad, like sick or anything. I was just bummed out.

PRACTITIONER: About what? [asking; open question]

PATIENT: About my friend. He's in trouble because I called the police on him. He was hurting me.

PRACTITIONER: Beating you up. [listening]

PATIENT: Kind of. He was slapping me and pushing me around, and I got scared.

PRACTITIONER: Has this happened before? [asking; closed question]

PATIENT: Yeah. He's hurt me before, but never this bad.

PRACTITIONER: It's getting worse, more serious, and that scares you. [listening]

PATIENT: He drinks, too, and he was drinking that night when he beat me up. I didn't know what he might do, so I called the cops.

Listening is not a passive process, but one in which the listener actively reflects back what the person has said. Good listening statements may continue the paragraph or make a guess about unspoken meaning.

Listening and Informing

Now the practitioner shifts to a mixture of listening and informing.

PRACTITIONER: You did the right thing. I see girls in here who didn't draw the line soon enough. [informing] You decided he'd gone too far. [listening]

PATIENT: I mean, we're still together, but he's mad at me.

PRACTITIONER: That must be scary. [listening]

PATIENT: You mean because he's mad at me?

PRACTITIONER: Well, I'm thinking that this guy was beating you up before, and now he's angry because you called the cops on him. That kind of cycle just tends to keep escalating. It isn't going to just disappear. [informing]

PATIENT: I know. I ought to break up with him and find somebody who treats me better.

PRACTITIONER: You've thought about it. [listening]

PATIENT: In fact, I was kind of looking around at the bar last night.

PRACTITIONER: I'd like you to take better care of yourself so I don't see you back here again. You've been allowing yourself to be in some pretty dangerous situations. [informing]

PATIENT: Yeah, well this is kind of a wake-up call.

PRACTITIONER: This got your attention, being strapped up here like this. You're thinking maybe it's time to wake up. [listening]

The preceding conversation clearly falls within the guiding style of MI that we have been describing, but other uses of the very same communication tools would not. Consider this example, also making use of asking, informing, and listening, but with a skeptical, directing style.

Practitioner: Doctor, nurse, physical therapist.
Setting: Cardiac rehabilitation or primary care.
Challenge: The patient leads a lifestyle that places him at risk for further problems.

PRACTITIONER: Hello, Mr. Bell. It's been 3 months since we did your bypass surgery, and I'm glad to see your test results. It looks like your heart is working well at this point. [informing] But I see from our records that you're still smoking. Is that right? [asking]

PATIENT: Yes, I am.

PRACTITIONER: Well, that's a problem, because, as you know, smoking is hard on your heart. [informing] You haven't quit yet? I'm sure you've been told about this? [asking]

PATIENT: It's just hard to quit. I've tried, really I have, but I just can't seem to do it.

PRACTITIONER: Can you see that places you at much higher risk for another heart attack? [asking]

PATIENT: I've been walking almost every day, like you told me.

PRACTITIONER: Almost every day. [listening] And yet you're still smoking. What about the diet we gave you? [asking]

PATIENT: I've still got it at home, and I'm trying to eat better.

PRACTITIONER: Aren't you using it? [asking]

PATIENT: Some, yes.

PRACTITIONER: Are you keeping to the diet? [asking]

PATIENT: I've tried some of the recipes, but I just don't enjoy them, and it takes a lot of work to cook that way. It's going to take me a while to get used to it.

PRACTITIONER: So you're making an effort, that's good. [listening] There are more changes I'd recommend if you want to keep healthy. You don't want to have another heart attack, do you?

PATIENT: No.

PRACTITIONER: Then you should try to quit smoking, use that diet we gave you, and get exercising as soon as possible. [informing]

This clinician is also asking, informing, and listening, but the tone of the consultation is distant from the guiding style of MI. It has an adversarial tone, with the clinician in the driver's seat telling the patient what to do and why to do it. Though asking questions, the clinician takes responsibility for making the change happen and does not seem to be interested in understanding the patient's own perspectives. The questions being asked do not elicit the patient's own motivations for behavior change. The clinician listens only minimally, just long enough to hear the patient's reply and then argue with it.

What is missing here is an honoring of the patient's autonomy, along with the collaborative, evocative style described in Chapter 1. It is within this "spirit" of motivational interviewing that the three communication tools come together to guide rather than badger, to encourage rather than shame, to negotiate rather than dictate. The guiding style is considerably more effective than lecturing when behavior change is needed, and it's also a lot more interesting and enjoyable for the clinician.

The three communication tools come together to guide rather than badger, to encourage rather than shame, to negotiate rather than dictate.

RESOLVING AMBIVALENCE

How does collaborative exploration of ambivalence start the process of behavior change moving? In talking about and reflecting on her or his own motivations for change, something clicks for the patient. You might think of it as the tipping of a balance or the flipping of a switch. In talking about why change is important, patients decide that it *really is* important. By voicing the good reasons to do it and how they might succeed, patients make change seem possible. There's a spark, and they quietly make the internal decision that behavior change may be worth the effort after all. They have literally talked themselves into doing it.

This is not usually accompanied by any fanfare. In fact, it may not be apparent to you that anything has happened. We have been through a guiding process with patients who seemed not to move at all, only to have them come back at the next visit and tell us they've made a change. One practitioner told us this:

In talking about why change is important, patients decide that it really is important. By voicing the good reasons to do it and how they might succeed, patients make change seem possible.

> "I had been seeing a patient who hadn't worked for years and was depressed. I had tried just about everything with him: medications, advice, encouraging him to exercise, get a job, and become active in social circles. Nothing seemed to help. He just seemed stuck, and I was feeling rather stuck and discouraged myself. Aware of how disheartened I was feeling, I looked at him and realized that he must be feeling all the more so. Not knowing what else to do, I offered a simple reflection: 'You must be feeling pretty fed up with all this.' All that he said was 'Yeah,' looking sullen as usual, and soon after that he left the office.
>
> "A few months later I saw him again for a minor medical problem, and I asked how he was getting on more generally. 'Wonderful!' he said brightly. 'I've got a job as a bus driver and I'm feeling great!' You could have knocked me over with a feather.
>
> " 'What happened?' I asked.
>
> " 'It was something that you said last time.' I had no idea what I had said that could possibly have had such an impact. 'When I left your office I realized that you were right: I was fed up with my life as it was, and I needed to do something about it. I saw an ad in the newspaper that the city was looking for bus drivers to train, and I called them up, and now I'm working a regular route and feeling great.' "

Listening for Commitment

Such surprises happen, but remember that there are also tangible cues to watch for as you talk with patients. There is, in particular, one reasonably reliable indicator that change is percolating: *commitment language*, as described in Chapter 5. It may emerge spontaneously as you practice MI ("I think I'll give this a try"), and there is also a way to assess whether the person is ready to move on. After giving the patient a summary of his or her own stated motivations for change (that DARN bouquet of flowers), ask a simple question the essence of which is, "So what are you thinking at this point? What are you going to do?"

There is a subtlety here in how you ask. When assessing commitment, use language such as:

"What *will* you do?"
"What are you *going* to do?"
"What are you *willing* to do?"
"What are you *prepared* to do?"

This is different from asking questions that merely elicit DARN statements:

"What do you *want* to do?" [desire]
or
"What *could* you do?" [ability]
or
"What do you *need* to do?" [need]

Consider this example, described to us by a colleague:

"I was treating a man whose wife was threatening to leave him and take the children away with her because of his drinking. He was a committed family man, had a good business, and all in all had experienced few of the ravages of overdrinking. His liver function tests were fairly normal except for raised GGT, which is often the first to go up in heavy drinkers. He was nevertheless drinking an astonishing amount on a daily basis, and it was causing real conflict at home. I tried motivational interviewing with him, and heard several change talk themes. His biggest concern, however, was loss of his wife and children, and as he talked about that possibility he volunteered, 'I guess that I just need to quit drinking.' After a few more minutes of listening, I offered him this summary:

'You certainly don't think of yourself as an alcoholic, or even a problem drinker. The main trouble has been at home, where you and your wife have been having a lot of arguments, mostly but not only about your drinking. It really shook you when she said she was thinking of leaving and taking the kids. Losing them, you said, would be the worst thing that could possibly happen to you. You were also surprised to see how much you were drinking when we added it all up. We also realized that you've been driving around legally intoxicated most mornings, given how long it takes to break down the alcohol that you drink at night. Most of all, though, you want to keep your family, and that's the biggest reason you came in. It sounds like you've decided that what you need to do is to stop drinking, at least for half a year or so, and see how you're feeling then. So is that what you want to do?'

" 'No,' he said.

"No? No? Damn! My thoughts were racing. I had just done my very best guiding summary, using exactly his own change talk, and led up to what he had told me was his plan. How could he now be saying no?

" 'No,' he said again. 'It's not what I *want* to do. It's what I'm *going* to do.'

"And he did."

The answer you are listening for is some level of commitment language as a signal of what is going on inside with regard to readiness. In essence, you are listening for what the patient is ready, willing, and able to do in the way of health behavior change. Don't push for it, though. Just give the patient opportunities to arrive at it. If the patient is not quite ready, pushing is just likely to evoke resistance. Instead, if you have a little more time, continue exploring DARN themes and leave the door open. If you will see the patient again, you can always resume the discussion at your next visit.

In essence, you are listening for what the patient is ready, willing, and able to do in the way of health behavior change. Don't push for it, though. Just give the patient opportunities to arrive at it.

You know that you are doing well with the guiding style when your patients happily keep talking to you, when they are expressing their own desire, ability, reasons, and need for behavior change. Done well, the guiding style opens patients to consider what they might do differently on behalf of their own health and to commit to taking such steps. Clinicians cannot make these decisions for patients; otherwise, many of us probably would. It is possible, however, to spend some time picking flowers in the meadow of ambivalence, to share the bouquet, and in the process to help patients find their own way into a healthier life.

Most likely, in considering this guiding style, you have thought about some of your patients who "just want to be told what to do." There certainly are such patients. They are scared and are ready, willing, and able to do whatever it takes to get better. What they want is not counseling but some clear direction about what they can do to restore or improve their health. It can be counterproductive to spend time discussing *why* to change with a patient who has already decided to do so. When someone says, "I need to stop smoking. How can I do it?" the appropriate response is advice about the most effective strategies. Clearly, that is what the patient is requesting. There are many other patients, however, who haven't yet reached that point of committed action. For every patient who says, "I plan to quit smoking," there are at least five other smokers who have not yet reached that point. At some level, patients know the changes they need to make in the interest of their health, but. . . .

CONCLUSION

MI is for helping that majority of your patients who are ambivalent to find within themselves their own motivations to change. In the next chapter we provide some case examples. We then turn to ways in which you can improve your MI skills (Chapter 9), and we end the book with attention focused on improving matters outside of the individual consultation (Chapter 10).

CHAPTER 8

Case Examples of a Guiding Style

In this chapter we offer some extended case studies drawn from our own clinical experience, to show what a guiding style might look like in everyday practice. If you like case examples, read on. If not, feel free to skip ahead to Chapter 9.

CASE 1: "MY STOMACH HURTS"

Setting: A general medical hospital ward.
Practitioner: Doctor, counselor, nurse, social worker, psychologist, addiction specialist.
Length of consultation: 4 minutes.
Challenge: A 52-year-old married woman is admitted to a hospital with abdominal pain and vomiting blood. The practitioner notices an elevated GGT value (a liver enzyme that is frequently elevated by excessive alcohol use) on the serum chemistry and suspects that drinking is involved. They have met once before. This woman might feel challenged and defensive if she were confronted about problem drinking. The prevention of readmission and promotion of health are worthy goals, but how does one raise the subject? The practitioner has just completed a review of her condition and continues . . .

PRACTITIONER: Well, you've had quite a shock, but I hope you are at least getting a rest here.

Open with an empathic statement.

PATIENT: Yes, thank you, I am feeling a little better. I don't get much rest at home—just rushing around in the car, go, go, go, like I'm on a mission, looking after the kids, the job, the food, you name it.

PRACTITIONER: You do a lot, and you get a lot done.

Listening.

PATIENT: Funny that you should say that. That's right, they call me supermom, and at work, I am the one who has to sort things out when it all goes crazy with stress and arguments about who's going to do this and that, and how we'll meet a deadline.

PRACTITIONER: I did want to ask you a little about your lifestyle. I'm not sure, but I wonder if there might be a connection here with what's going on in your stomach. Could we talk for a few minutes about this?

Brief agenda setting; raises the topic of lifestyle in general. Asking permission.

PATIENT: No, that's OK. Superwoman has landed in trouble. What are you thinking?

First hint of change talk.

PRACTITIONER: I'm not sure. Diet, alcohol, running around too much? I'm not sure. You'll be the best judge of this, but it sounds like you lead a pretty hectic life.

Only gentle informing. Promotes autonomy and returns to her story about her lifestyle.

PATIENT: Hectic's not the word.

PRACTITIONER: You must enjoy living in the fast lane.

Listening; a guess.

PATIENT: I do like getting things done. It's kind of a buzz, zooming from one thing to the next.

PRACTITIONER: Do you ever move over into the slow lane?

Asking: a guiding question, making use of the driving metaphor.

PATIENT: It's hard—it's no joke, there's so much to do, I just don't relax.

She seems much more emotional.

PRACTITIONER: What things do you do to take care of yourself?

Asking; a guiding question, seeking to understand where alcohol may fit in.

PATIENT: At night when the kids are in bed, sometimes I watch movies and open a bottle of wine. That's my time. The only time I get, really.

She raises the topic of drinking within a normal everyday context.

PRACTITIONER: That helps you slow down, maybe relax a little at night.

Listening.

PATIENT: And sometimes on weekends I go out with my friends and we have a few drinks.

PRACTITIONER: Drinking is a way you relax. Tell me, what do you know about how alcohol can affect the stomach?

Listening. Information exchange: Elicit by asking what she knows.

PATIENT: It can make you hungry, like an appetizer. Do you think that's what's causing this? Is that what you're saying?

A little defensive.

PRACTITIONER: It might be part of what's happening. I noticed on your blood tests that one value was up in the abnormal range, a liver function test that is often elevated by alcohol.

Information exchange: Provide.

PATIENT: Oh great! The one thing I do for myself, and you want to take it away.

Defensive.

PRACTITIONER: I don't want to jump to conclusions, and in any case, it's your choice what to do. I can't decide that for you.

Avoids premature focus and emphasizes choice and autonomy.

PATIENT: I just want a normal life. I want my stomach to stop hurting, and I want to get out of here.

PRACTITIONER: You've had a pretty rough ride lately. And I want those things for you, too—a life that works for you and doesn't put you back here in the hospital.

Listening and encouragement.

PATIENT: Now what about that blood test you mentioned? That scares me a little.

Question gives permission to inform.

PRACTITIONER: It's one that often goes up when a person is drinking more than the body can handle. You're pretty slim, which means that a little alcohol goes a long way. Also women don't break down alcohol in the liver as well as men do.

Information exchange: Provide.

PATIENT: So are you telling me I need to cut back?

PRACTITIONER: It's up to you, but it seems like that's what your body is telling you. Also, a stressful life can be hard on the stomach, and adding alcohol on top of that can cause problems.

Emphasizing choice and autonomy. Informing.

PATIENT: How does that work?

Question gives permission to inform.

PRACTITIONER: Alcohol itself irritates the gullet and stomach lining. Have you ever drunk straight liquor and felt the burn?

Informing.

PATIENT: Sure.

PRACTITIONER: That burning is alcohol's effect. It also releases stomach acid, which is why it can increase your

Informing.

appetite, and that can add to the problem if your stomach is already weak from stress, and you can wind up with ulcers. What are you thinking at this point?	*Information exchange: elicit her personal interpretation.*
PATIENT: I don't want an ulcer. Do you think that's what I have?	*Change talk—reason to do something.*
PRACTITIONER: It could be. There are tests that can look into this. If it is, what do you think you will do?	*Open question.*
PATIENT: I assume you'll have some medicine for me to take. But I guess I also need to cut down my drinking, even if I don't have an ulcer.	*Change talk (need).*
PRACTITIONER: How hard would that be for you?	*Guiding question—looking for change talk (ability).*
PATIENT: Not hard, really. I'd just have to find another way to relax.	*Change talk—ability.*
PRACTITIONER: So you *could* cut down your drinking if you decided to. Even quit drinking?	*Reflective listening. Guiding question.*
PATIENT: I'm not so sure.	
PRACTITIONER: So why would you want to cut down or quit?	*Guiding question.*
PATIENT: For my health! It sounds like I might be eating a hole in my stomach, and my liver is getting abnormal. I think it's time.	*Change talk.*
PRACTITIONER: Seems like it to me, too. What will you do?	*Asking for commitment.*
PATIENT: I can just not keep any alcohol in the house to tempt me. I think that's what I'll probably do.	*Change talk. First indication of commitment.*

CASE 2: PROMOTING SAFE SEX

This next scenario occurs all over the world. In places where the rates of HIV/AIDS are high, the practitioner is faced with a health promotion challenge that could be a life-or-death matter not just for the patients but also for those with whom they have sexual contact.

Setting: A busy primary care clinic in an area with high HIV/AIDS rates.
Practitioner: Doctor, nurse.
Length of consultation: 5 minutes.
Challenge: A man comes in with a sexually transmitted bacterial infection and is examined and given antibiotics. The practitioner wonders about him being HIV-positive and about the possibility of multiple partners and the value of his using condoms. This man is in his 40s, he's single, most often unemployed, and lives with a wider extended family on the outskirts of a large city. The practitioner uses mostly information exchange to raise concerns about unprotected sex.

PRACTITIONER: OK, I think we'll get this infection under control if you take this medicine faithfully for the next 10 days. Will you do that?	*Asking for commitment.*
PATIENT: Sure.	
PRACTITIONER: Good! It's important to finish it all. I wonder if it would be all right for me to talk with you for a few more minutes. I'm interested not only in helping you deal with medical problems but also in keeping you healthy. Would that be all right?	*Asking permission.*
PATIENT: OK, sure. What do you want to talk about?	
PRACTITIONER: It's part of my job to talk with you about avoiding all sorts of infections, including HIV/AIDS. What do you already know about HIV?	*Agenda setting, raising a difficult subject. Asking (information exchange: Elicit).*

PATIENT: If you get it, you die. But I'm pretty careful. I just didn't use a condom this one time. Just one of those things that happens.

PRACTITIONER: Good! So usually you do use a condom. It just happens sometimes that you don't, and you caught this infection.

Affirming.
Reflective listening.

PATIENT: Bad luck, I guess. I just met this girl, and she didn't look unhealthy. Who knows where she got it from.

PRACTITIONER: Makes you wonder. Maybe she didn't know either.

Listening.

PATIENT: So I got unlucky and got it from her. It happens.

PRACTITIONER: You've mentioned that several times now—that it's just a matter of luck or chance. These infections just go around and around.

Listening.

PATIENT: Yeah, see, I've never had a problem like this before. I have this one steady girlfriend, and this was just a one-night thing with this other girl.

PRACTITIONER: I hope you don't mind my asking you about this. I really don't want to make you uncomfortable by asking about your personal life, but I do care about your health.

Asking permission and respecting autonomy.

PATIENT: No, it's OK.

PRACTITIONER: So you had unprotected sex with this one girl, and you have a steady girlfriend. What kind of protection do you use with your regular girlfriend?

Listening.

Asking.

PATIENT: We always use a condom, or most of the time, anyway.

PRACTITIONER: Sometimes you don't, but most of the time you do. OK. Now, tell me what you know about how worse infections like HIV spread.	*Listening.* *Asking (Information exchange: Elicit).*
PATIENT: Oh, God! You've got to be joking. Do you think I have AIDS?	
PRACTITIONER: I have no idea at all whether you might have picked up HIV along the way. We can test you to find out while you are here today, if you want. What I'm asking, though, is what you know about how people do get HIV and AIDS.	*Avoiding premature focus.* *Acknowledging choice.* *More eliciting.*
PATIENT: Well, you get unlucky, and you get very sick, I've seen it, but I don't lead that kind of life, sleeping around with dirty girls.	
PRACTITIONER: I don't know if this will make sense or matter to you, but I can tell you that infections like HIV often spread quietly among all sorts of people who look healthy for many years before they get sick. The infection can be passed without either person knowing it. What do you think about that?	*Asking permission.* *Information exchange: Provide.* *Information exchange: Elicit.*
PATIENT: I just had this one night with a new girl!	
PRACTITIONER: And you're really not at all worried about that.	*Listening, continuing the paragraph (no tone of sarcasm).*
PATIENT: Well, maybe I have to be more careful.	*First change talk.*
PRACTITIONER: In what way?	*Asking.*
PATIENT: Like I guess I shouldn't sleep around too much, and be sure to use condoms if I do.	*Change talk.*

PRACTITIONER: It is certainly true that having just one partner does decrease your risk. So do condoms, if you use them all the time. How important is this for you?

Informing.

Asking for change talk.

PATIENT: I don't know.

PRACTITIONER: Let me ask you this. On a scale from 1 to 10, where 1 is not at all important and 10 is extremely important, how important would you say it is for you to use condoms every time, even with your steady girlfriend?

Using an importance ruler.

PATIENT: Probably 8 or 9.

Change talk.

PRACTITIONER: OK—you have a little doubt, but it's very important to you, for your health, to protect yourself. And you're protecting other people, too.

Reflective listening.

PATIENT: Yeah, I hope I didn't give this infection to my girlfriend. She'd go crazy.

PRACTITIONER: Yes, infections can spread quickly and quietly among people who look and feel perfectly healthy. So you've had unprotected sex with your girlfriend after this other girl.

Informing.

Listening.

PATIENT: Yeah, well, we used a condom, but they don't always work, right?

PRACTITIONER: They're not 100% effective, but they do give you good protection. If she develops any symptoms, I can treat her, too.

Informing.

PATIENT: I just hope that girl didn't have HIV.

PRACTITIONER: Me, too. It just takes one time, as you see. It takes a while to get the results, but the test for HIV is easy. Shall we do it?

Informing.

Asking.

PATIENT: Oh, man. I don't know. I don't think it's very likely.

PRACTITIONER: Maybe not. You really can't tell from looking at someone, and people can be healthy for a long time before they get sick. There is much better treatment available these days, and knowing early on if one is positive or not can help plan treatment.

Resisting the temptation to argue. Informing.

PATIENT: I guess I ought to know.

Change talk.

PRACTITIONER: OK, good. I'll draw a blood sample and make an appointment for you to come back, when we can have a discussion about what the test means and that sort of thing. So to summarize, you have been using condoms most of the time but not all the time. You picked up this infection from one time when you didn't, and you hope you haven't already passed it on to your girlfriend. It's unpleasant to think about, but you want to be tested for HIV so you know. And what about using condoms?

Offering a short summary.

Asking for commitment.

PATIENT: I need to use them all the time, I guess.

Change talk.

PRACTITIONER: How confident are you that you'll succeed?

Asking for commitment.

PATIENT: Yeah, I'll try. It's hard sometimes.

Moderate commitment. "I'll try" bespeaks doubt about ability.

PRACTITIONER: Good for you! I'm glad. And maybe when you come back we can talk a little about the times when it's harder to use protection.

Affirming. Setting the stage for discussion to increase ability in more difficult circumstances.

CASE 3: A MATTER OF THE HEART

Setting: An outpatient cardiovascular rehabilitation clinic. This same discussion might also take place in a primary care clinic or an inpatient setting.

Practitioner: Nurse, doctor, occupational therapist, physical therapist, counselor, psychologist.

Length of consultation: About 20 minutes.

Challenge: The patient had a heart attack 12 weeks ago and is being seen for follow-up. The practitioner might want to encourage change in many interrelated behaviors: smoking, exercise, diet, or alcohol consumption. The patient has a cheerful disposition, works as a clerk, enjoys life (with cigarettes, alcohol, and good food!) and is surrounded by a busy family life, including two adolescent children.

PRACTITIONER: Can we spend some time now talking about how you are doing at home, because all sorts of things can affect the health of your heart. It's not just the medication that matters. Would that be OK?

Asking permission.

Start of agenda setting.

PATIENT: Yes, I suppose I'm due for a lecture about what a bad boy I am and how I have to stop everything I enjoy. (*Laughs.*)

PRACTITIONER: Well, actually that is not what I'm going to do. I promise. It's totally up to you what you want to do about your health. It sounds, though, like you were hoping the pills would do the whole trick for you.

She avoids the temptation to argue for lifestyle change, emphasizes autonomy, offers a listening statement.

PATIENT: Well, you said that I'm making a good recovery and that the medicine seems to be the right one.

PRACTITIONER: Yes, indeed, I'm pleased with how you have recovered from the bypass surgery. What it comes down to now is what you want to do among all

Informing and agenda setting.

the things that can reduce your chances of another heart attack and help you have a good quality of life. I could give you some facts and figures that might surprise and encourage you, but to start with let's take a look at the bigger picture of your life and see what makes sense for you.

PATIENT: All right. What do you think I should do first?

An invitation.

PRACTITIONER: That's really up to *you* to decide. You're in charge of your own life. We could talk about exercise, smoking, diet, monitoring your blood pressure, decreasing stress, meditating, or just being faithful about taking your medications. What makes sense to you?

She declines the initial invitation, emphasizes autonomy, and sets an agenda by offering a menu of possible topics for the patient to choose from.

PATIENT: Well, where do you think I should start?

Gives permission to inform and advise.

PRACTITIONER: I do have some information I can give you, if you want, and my own opinion about what changes might help most. But you probably already know the score. What's your guess about what I'll say?

She offers to give information and advice but tries just once more to elicit it from him first.

PATIENT: I'll bet you start with telling me to quit smoking.

And it succeeds.

PRACTITIONER: Good guess! I do think that quitting smoking is the one thing you could do that would likely have the biggest and quickest impact on your risk of dying prematurely. But what do you think about that?

Affirming.
Informing.

A key question in the service of guiding.

PATIENT: Smoking is completely part of my life.

PRACTITIONER: Smoking is a tough one for you—a hard place to start.

Reflective listening.

PATIENT: Well, I know it's bad for me, and I did ask you what you think.	*Change talk.*
PRACTITIONER: You've got your own feelings about smoking, though, no matter what anyone else thinks.	*Listening statement. Avoids temptation to take up the antismoking side.*
PATIENT: I feel like, look, it's just not going to happen right now. I'm having a hard enough time getting back on my feet.	
PRACTITIONER: Quitting smoking is just too hard for you right now, and you have other priorities.	*Listening. She resists temptation to take up the pro side of quitting.*
PATIENT: Right, I've got to get back to work now, for a few hours a week at least. And I want to get my stress level down while I get back to normal activities.	*Change talk.*
PRACTITIONER: That's your top priority right now—to get back to work and manage your stress.	*Listening.*
PATIENT: Well, I want to get back to work. But to be perfectly honest, I do sometimes feel like I could have another attack any moment and whack, I'd be gone.	*Change talk.*
PRACTITIONER: So you feel like you just need to rest right now.	*Listening.*
PATIENT: Not exactly. I'm not just resting all the time. I'm moving around, doing this and that, trying to get a little exercise.	*The practitioner's guess was not quite right, and the patient corrects it.*
PRACTITIONER: You're trying to get the balance right.	*Listening—trying again.*
PATIENT: Yes, that's it. A balance.	

PRACTITIONER: So what you've told me so far is that you're taking your medications, resting up a bit, but also trying to get some exercise, which is good for your heart. You already knew that quitting smoking is one of the biggest things you could do for your heart, but that just seems impossible right now. And you're eager to get back to work, at least part time, as soon as possible, and get your life back in balance. Did I miss anything?	*Collecting summary, emphasizing change talk themes.*
PATIENT: Well, not *back* in balance exactly. I don't think I ever had a very good balance before this heart attack, and that was part of the problem. I'm just not sure where to start.	*Change talk.*
PRACTITIONER: You did mention decreasing your stress level, too. How might you do that?	*Asking.*
PATIENT: I think this gives me a chance to do that. I think I need to start turning some things over to other people. I'm the kind who always thinks, "If you want something done right, do it yourself." Then I'm stressed out with how much I have to do.	
PRACTITIONER: It could help to take some things off your plate.	*Listening.*
PATIENT: Now there you go with lecturing me about diet! (*Laughs.*) No, that's what I need to do—trust the people around me to do their jobs, and focus on what's really important. I can't change everything at once.	*Change talk.*
PRACTITIONER: If you could do just that much—reduce the burden of what you have to do—that would help.	*Listening.*

A key moment has been reached in the consultation, a crossroads of sorts. What would you say next? This man has said a lot already, and it is heartfelt material. Suppose you have a little longer to listen. Where would you go next? If you look at what he's said, you could focus on (1) his gradual return to work, (2) more specific plans about exercise, (3) when he might be ready to quit smoking, (4) stress management, (5) how to delegate responsibilities he has been carrying, or (6) pick up on the passing invitation to talk about diet. Or you could go off in an entirely different direction. Reflecting on any one of these themes will focus the discussion and lead off in a particular direction. This is what we mean by listening in the service of guiding. It's your choice, and it makes a difference what you choose.

As this example continues, the practitioner does try a different direction, responding to an intuition that this patient doesn't seem to have something to live *for*, except perhaps his work. Its an exploration of core values. Why then, the practitioner wonders, would he *want* to make healthy changes? What would motivate him to do so?

PRACTITIONER: You know, I really like your idea that this heart attack is an opportunity for you to make some changes and to consider what is really important. Could I ask you, what are the most important things in your life? What are you living *for*?	*Affirming.* *Asking permission.* *Open question.*
PATIENT: Oh, uh, that's a good question. I like my work. My family—I want to see that my kids get started off in the right direction. In fact, I'd like to be there for my grandchildren, if we have them. That looks like fun.	
PRACTITIONER: Your work, your kids, maybe grandchildren some day. What else? What really *matters* to you?	*Listening.* *Open question.*
PATIENT: I thought about that in the hospital bed. Since I'm alive, what do I want to do with the life I have left?	
PRACTITIONER: Yes. What is it you want to do?	*Open question.*

PATIENT: Help others, my family, and be there for them, if you see what I mean?

PRACTITIONER: That's what's really important for you, being around for a reason, and for helping others. *Listening.*

PATIENT: To think about someone besides myself. To remind me what I have to be grateful for.

PRACTITIONER: You know, you kind of light up when you talk about this. *Listening.*

PATIENT: Well, I've been out of touch, and there's lots I can do for my family and other people, even in a club, which I used to volunteer for. *Change talk.*

PRACTITIONER: We've talked about a lot so far, and you're developing a pretty good list of things you can do to make your life longer and happier. Is there anything else from that list I gave you earlier that you'd like to talk about? *Summary. She decides to change direction and see where behavior change might fit into this bigger picture. Returns to agenda setting.*

PATIENT: Maybe diet and exercise.

PRACTITIONER: What concerns you about that? *Asking a guiding question.*

PATIENT: I'm not concerned, really. I'm just wondering what I should be doing in that area. *The practitioner chose a word, "concerned," that didn't quite fit.*

PRACTITIONER: There's quite a lot of things you *could* do. Making small, gradual changes in what you eat. Increasing fruits and vegetables to five or so a day. Building some modest exercise into your regular daily routine. *Offering a menu of options.* Would any of that be workable for you? *Asking.*

PATIENT: Well, maybe the exercise thing, but I don't really want to go to a gym or anything like that. I don't want to have another heart attack! *Change talk.*

PRACTITIONER: Adding some kind of exercise might be OK for you, but definitely not the gym yet. What kind of exercise do you get at the moment?

Listening.

Guiding question.

PATIENT: Not enough. I just do a bit of walking a few times a week. Sometimes when I do that I get these feelings in my chest, and I worry I'm pushing myself too hard.

PRACTITIONER: That's really a common worry, and our experience suggests that as long as people do things gradually, no harm comes their way. We could help you develop a gradual, step-by-step program to increase your exercise. If you'd feel better about it, you could even use the facilities here, and we can monitor your heart rate at first to make sure it's safe.

Informing.

PATIENT: That sounds good. But mostly I think walking is what will work for me. I could do more of that.

Change talk.

PRACTITIONER: And that's what's important—to find what you can do that works for you and fits with your normal life. And if you do have any of these feelings while you're walking on your own, just stop, rest, and manage them as we've discussed before.

Informing.

PATIENT: OK. Maybe I'll take you up on a little monitoring while I exercise here.

Change talk.

PRACTITIONER: Fine! We can set that up. Well, we've covered a lot of ground today in a short time. Help me remember it all. First and foremost, you are choosing to think about this heart attack as an opportunity for you to make some good changes in your life and to get your priorities straight. You are

Closing summary.

She puts the positive motivations up front.

devoted to your work and also to your family, and you want to be around to help your children and maybe grandchildren get a good start in life. You're also feeling a desire to get more involved in helping others, at home and in other places like the club. To do that, there are some lifestyle changes that you're planning to make. One of these, as you gradually get back to work, is to decrease the volume of work that you take on and perhaps find some other ways to decrease your stress and get your life in balance. Smoking is something we'll talk about later, because right now that seems too difficult to change. If you decide to tackle that later, I have some ways to help you with it. You're already doing a good job taking your medications, and you're doing at least a little walking, which you want to increase. We can set you up for some modest monitored exercise here—we can do that as you leave today. That sounds like a lot of change right there. I look forward to seeing you over the months ahead to see how you're doing with this and help in any way I can with these or other changes. Is that what you are going to do? Anything I missed?

Then she talks about specific changes they have discussed.

She accepts and acknowledges the situation with smoking, leaving the door open.

Affirming.

Asking for commitment.

PATIENT: That sounds about right. I feel like I'm headed in the right direction, like there is something I can do.

Change talk.

CONCLUSION

There's no single "correct" way to conduct a consultation, so if you have found places where you might have done things differently, take this as a stimulus to be creative in your own consultations. Our intention here was to illustrate the underlying style of MI, difficult when using only the written word, and to indicate where relevant skills and strategies such as listening and agenda setting were used. The next chapter turns to some of the more subtle things to look out for as you refine your skills in MI.

CHAPTER 9

Getting Better at Guiding

GETTING USED TO GUIDING

Guiding is not just about what one says to patients; it is also about how one *is* with them. This was nicely illustrated in a recent workshop with prison officers. The simulations were going well enough with the participants standing up, but when it came to a sequence of guiding, one of them announced, "I can't do this standing up. I need to sit down with this person."

A common observation made by practitioners is "it doesn't feel natural." Indeed, this way of working with patients is often very different from prior practice, from following the righting reflex of just directing someone what to do and why. Try out this style in easier situations first, when time feels manageable and your patient seems engaged. As you become more proficient, you can move on to more difficult challenges.

Try out this guiding style in easier situations first, when time feels manageable and your patient seems engaged.

It can take a while for the guiding style to begin feeling natural. It's a bit like learning to drive a car. On your first time behind the wheel, you were probably highly self-conscious, and understandably so. You drove slowly, with heightened awareness, trying not to stray into the next lane. You had to focus on tasks inside the car yet also had to keep an eye out to make sure you weren't about to run someone over. You had to think about where you were going and attend to so many new tasks simultaneously. But you didn't give up learning to drive just because it didn't feel natural at first.

As you become more comfortable with the component skills of any new endeavor—whether driving or guiding—you do not have to think about them so consciously. The skills become mostly automatic, and you can concentrate instead on where you are going, how you will get there, and what you will do when you arrive. Learning is like that, and learning the guiding style is no different. At first you are self-conscious, particularly when being observed. Are you asking an open or closed question? Are you reflectively listening? Focusing directly on the guidelines is necessary at first, but it also keeps you from seeing where you are going. In time, comfort with these skills gives rise to other freedoms. It becomes easier to notice other things that are also important in skillful guiding.

Think now about the role of the driving instructor. He or she might take the wheel in an emergency, but, in general, the task is to encourage the learner to make progress with as little intervention from the instructor as possible. This is similar to your role in guiding the patient. It is the patient who has to do the changing; you let go of control more and more.

As you become more comfortable with the specific techniques involved in MI, your attention is freed to monitor the guiding process itself. Your attention can switch between three aspects of the consultation: your relationship with the patient, what he or she is saying, and where you might go next. With practice, you can move between these roles with relative ease. Here are examples of these three processes.

Watching the Relationship

Your awareness of the relationship is a barometer of skill and good outcome. Keeping a keen eye on the relationship will help you to decide where and how to proceed. Check in with yourself by asking: How are we getting on in this discussion? How is the patient reacting? Is she or he comfortable, or frightened, perhaps? Am I pushing this person too hard? Am I being genuine and frank?

Staying in the Present

Psychotherapists refer to being "in the moment" with the patient. There are important periods when your own aspirations, feelings, and personal reactions are put to one side and you focus your full attention on the patient's experience. The more you are able to do this, the more effective your guiding response is likely to be, whether it is a listening reflection, a well-chosen question, or offering important information.

Some commentators say that this attentiveness is in itself a powerful nonspecific route to healing, leading to an empathic relationship that frees the person to change. When patients sense this clear understanding of their experience from you, things begin to happen, and change often follows. Acceptance of a patient's experience is not the same as agreeing. It is relatively free of judgment—whether positive or negative—and therein lies the potential for you to be a good guide.

Acceptance of a patient's experience is not the same as agreeing. It is relatively free of judgment—whether positive or negative—and therein lies the potential for you to be a good guide.

Looking Ahead

Sometimes your attention moves ahead to where the consultation is going, how it will end, and, indeed, what it will be like when the patient steps back into everyday life. With increasing skill, you find that you are able to consider the route ahead and watch for obstacles, often during short pauses in the conversation. At these moments, you can learn to find the short cuts, the kind of guiding question or reflective listening statement that gets you closest to what is helpful for the patient and saves time, as well.

As you trust patients to take control, you give them more room to talk, and this gives you freedom to concentrate on where you are going. This letting go of control is not an all-or-nothing matter. One clinician emerged from a simulated exercise and said, "I get it. There's no need to worry about control. Instead of push this way and shove that way, it's just nudge, listen, and summarize, nudge, listen, and summarize. . . ." After a while you realize that you actually don't lose your capacity to encourage change; quite the opposite. Guiding then begins to feel natural.

"I get it. There's no need to worry about control. Instead of push this way and shove that way, it's just nudge, listen, and summarize, nudge, listen, and summarize. . . ."

"But I Can't Let Go of Responsibility"

Many a discussion about the skill involved in guiding returns to the subject of responsibility. "It's all very well," someone usually says, "but I've got a job to do. I must raise these subjects. It's my responsibility. I can't just let them decide for themselves!" This can lead into the trap of "either–or thinking," of the falsely limiting choice between directing or following. "I either tell them what to do [direct], or leave them to work it out by themselves [follow]." Sitting in the middle ground between directing and following means taking responsibility for the structure and direction of the consultation *and* encouraging patients to come up with their own solutions to behavior-change problems. As you get better at guiding, you will be able to sense when it is the right time to move on in the consultation, to summarize and shift direction, or even to adopt a directing style and consider another topic. When you are listening to patients, try to focus not on what is happening to the time but on how you might capture your understanding of their dilemma in a useful way. Brief reflections or longer summaries are particularly useful here. Often, you can emerge from a few minutes of this activity with both parties clearer about the way ahead. Seen in this light, you are the guardian of the journey as a whole, much like the driving instructor, but the patient is the guardian of motives and strategies for changing behavior. A good guide promotes freedom of choice and provides high-quality support and advice when needed.

Sitting in the middle ground between directing and following means taking responsibility for the structure and direction of the consultation and encouraging patients to come up with their own solutions to behavior-change problems.

OVERCOMING OBSTACLES

Obstacles to guiding are everywhere! As you become more skillful, you develop an ability to overcome them not through forceful or clever effort but by clear agenda setting, curiosity, and a genuine concern and respect for patients' ability to clarify what's best for them, a fertile ground for the use of listening skills. New avenues open up, and things feel easier.

One of the origins of MI came from the realization that when things are difficult in the conversation, there is often an unproductive tendency to blame the patient. When rapport is undermined, which invariably is the case when things get tough, what can you do to repair this and return to the kind of constructive conversation described previously?

The following discussion focuses on common challenges from three overlapping perspectives: that of the patient, that of the practitioner, and the relationship between the two. Sometimes the way the patient reacts (e.g., defensiveness) and your response (e.g., irritation) provides a clear signal that all is not well. Responding flexibly and creatively is a challenge that can bring rewards fairly immediately.

The Patients: Their Struggles

Patients can feel bewildered, frustrated, defensive, passive, and overwhelmed by circumstances. Talking about change can be difficult, and a temptation to label and blame the person can undermine your best intentions to use a guiding style. Consider the following common scenarios.

"I Can't See Why I Need to Change"

"They are in complete denial" is a phrase that is used widely across many health care settings. Patients apparently shut down when faced with efforts to encourage them to consider change or to consider the seriousness of their situation. If you use a directing style in this situation by arguing for change, progress can freeze entirely. The more you push someone into looking at something, the more he or she will resist and defend him- or herself. If you come alongside him or her, and clarify what *is* important to him or her in some form of agenda setting (see Chapter 4), the denial will often subside, and you might be able to make progress. Denial is not a fixed property inside someone but a reaction that arises during communication between two people in a particular circumstance, often when someone's self-esteem is under threat.

Denial is not a fixed property inside someone but a reaction that arises during communication between two people in a particular circumstance, often when someone's self-esteem is under threat.

Refusal to consider change can arise even when you use a guiding style, perhaps because you have prematurely focused on behavior change. Someone who has just had surgery or an acute medical crisis might feel so preoccupied that he or she does not want or cannot absorb even skillful and well-meant efforts to raise the subject of behavior change. This is common in cardiac rehabilitation, diabetes, and the care of all long-term conditions. Something else is of greater concern, or the patient's experience of illness lies hidden behind whatever conversation unfolds. Some patients with asthma, for example, resist efforts to encourage the use of prophylactic medicine because they do not share your view about exactly what the problem is. Your use of listening is the key to unlocking this impasse. Five minutes of seeking clarity can lay open the path to behavior change and prevent wasted time and visits.

"I Can See What You Mean, but . . . "

You get so far, and they back off. A moment is reached when patients' words veer away from talk about change and a voice of defensiveness expresses precisely the opposite. Subtle moment-to-moment shifts in willingness to consider change are normal and common when a patient is feeling ambivalent. At this point just a slight overemphasis on your part on encouraging change can lead to a corresponding counterreaction. If you are prepared for this and accept it as completely normal, you can stay calm enough to respond appropriately—for example, by reflecting both sides of the person's ambivalence. Patience and acceptance of this seemingly irrational process are usually most helpful.

Subtle moment-to-moment shifts in willingness to consider change are normal and common when a patient is feeling ambivalent.

"Just Tell Me What You Think I Should Do!"

Some patients look up to you for the answer. Perhaps that is the way people in a particular neighborhood, culture, or language or age group seem to use health care services. If they do not seem keen to come up with their own ideas, it is quite feasible to switch from eliciting solutions from them to providing information and advice, all within a guiding style. You simply offer one or more suggestions and use a guiding question to check that this makes sense, for example, "How will this work for you?"

"I Really Can't Cope at All"

A patient is lonely, overwhelmed by poor housing, has no spare money, has a chronic health problem such as diabetes, and now you want to raise the possibility of behavior change. All the dangers of not listening lie before you. Conveying your understanding of his or her predicament and affirming his or her strengths in coping with these circumstances can provide the platform for a more focused agenda-setting process that considers ways of enhancing control of his or her situation. A discussion of genuinely helpful behavior change often follows.

Trouble in the consultation about behavior change often goes both ways. It is the meeting place for a marriage of sorts between your aspirations and those of the patient. We turn now to what you may feel in the guiding consultation, sometimes an obstacle to progress as well.

The Practitioner: Your Feelings

It is very common to feel different things about different patients. You like some, and others less so. You can feel concerned, frustrated, annoyed, or even outraged by their predicaments, their attitudes, or the pressure you are under to undertake different tasks. The calmness at the heart of guiding is not always easy to achieve.

You cannot be expected to be in a state of perfect calm in the midst of busy everyday practice; neither can you become a psychotherapist, practiced in the art of monitoring feelings and their effects on the relationship with the patient. Yet feelings can run high, and your own emotional state affects the process and outcome of the consultation. One senior physician we worked with threw into a conversation the following phrase: "If I work on automatic pilot, and I am even a little bit stressed, I produce tired, automatic responses." Then he explained about the importance of awareness and acceptance of what one is feeling: "After so many years at this, I've learned to check on what I am feeling at any point in time. It's funny, but I know my moods. If I realize I am too stressed out to really help a patient, I don't get worked up about it, I just accept it. Then I settle down, and I feel more flexible."

Aspirations for Behavior Change

Some of the most powerful forces affecting patient progress toward change are your own thoughts and feelings about what might be good for the patient. We have called these your *aspirations for patient behavior change* (ABCs). They are common and perfectly normal, but if they are allowed to dominate the consultation, they can make it difficult to honor the autonomy of patients to decide what is best for themselves.

If your aspirations for patient behavior change (ABCs) are allowed to dominate the consultation, they can make it difficult to honor the autonomy of patients to decide what is best for themselves.

You raise the subject of behavior change, and you want to succeed. *Wanting* someone to change, however, comes in many colors, and strong feelings can prevail: hope, enthusiasm, determination, irritation, anger, and even hopelessness can take their own toll on your well-being and skillfulness. Mindfulness about how you feel before and during the consultation might provide the key to doing a better job. Consider these examples, in which most practitioners would *want* the patient to change:

- She is working as a prostitute to feed her heroin addiction, and she is about to lose custody of her child.
- If he does not cut down his liquid intake soon, his heart will begin to fail, and he will die.

Practitioners often have a silent internal monologue going while in conversation with patients such as these. The monologue often contains what could be called practitioner change talk. "I want to help him get to the bottom of this, and turn things around" (desire). "I think I can make a difference here" (ability). "She really must change because that child is going to suffer terribly" (reasons). "I must raise the subject" (need). "I'm going to give her the extra time she needs now" (commitment). These aspirations can reflect deeply held personal values: "This is why I came into this job, to help people like this turn their lives around." They can also have negative aspects: "Oh, no, the situation just seems hopeless. I don't know where to begin."

Health care is replete with people in predicaments that practitioners want to change, thus setting up a conflict with practitioners' simultaneous desire to respect patients' freedom to make their minds up for themselves. Here is an example of how this conflict appears in a conversation between colleagues:

Practitioner A: "I want to get this patient to change her diet so we can lower her blood sugar levels."
Practitioner B: "But you can't *get* her to do anything. It's up to her."

It is not uncommon for a practitioner to hold both of these views simultaneously. Your aspirations for behavior change are high, *and* you also respect the patient's freedom to make up his or her own mind. These are not necessarily incompatible. They are part of the delicate challenge that characterizes the behavior-change consultation. An adept and sure-footed rock-climbing guide might watch the struggle of the climber and very much want him or her to succeed but will also be very mindful that he cannot do it for him or her. Allowing the climber to find his or her own way within clear safety parameters and accepting the outcome with patience and respect is what makes for a good working relationship between them.

There are also situations in which these ABCs are not highly charged and you do not really care whether the person changes his or her behavior or not; this situation is sometimes called a *position of equipoise.*

- "This is tricky, whether to use this medication or not. It's his de cision, the arguments for and against are finely balanced."
- "I can see problems looming with her feet, but she has other priorities in the control of her diabetes. I don't mind if we don't talk about feet right now."

Just as you can view a patient's readiness to change on a continuum, you could consider your desire for the behavior change along similar lines, say from 1–10, where 1 means that you are in equipoise and 10 means that you feel very strongly about the value of change.

How might this help you in the consultation? Simply being aware that you have high ABCs should help you to back off. The goal is to avoid letting the ABCs dominate the exchange with the patient. If you do not succeed, you might fall into any of a number of traps. Here are some examples.

ABCs and Some Common Traps

The stronger your feelings about wanting the patient to change, the more mindful you might need to be about your own behavior. There is nothing wrong with wanting and hoping for behavior change in your patients, but strong ABCs can mislead you into the righting reflex and other difficulties. Monitoring how you are feeling is the first step. Then you might want to be careful not to fall into a pattern of responding that strays some distance from guiding. Here are some examples.

Monitoring how strongly you feel about patient behavior change is the first step in avoiding difficulties.

DESCENDING INTO DIRECTING

Sometimes you choose a directing style not because you sense that the patient expects this but because of your feelings about how important it is for him or her to change. You might be feeling under time pressure or simply so keen to promote change that you adopt a directing style. The outcome is some distance from guiding. This can happen in the opening seconds of a discussion:

PRACTITIONER: [feeling quite determined] Now I've been meaning to ask you, have you done anything about your smoking, because it's a big worry for your health.

PATIENT: [shutting down immediately] Well, I never lasted long when I quit before, so I am just getting on with my life.

PERSUADING TOO HARD

Your desire to encourage change can lead you into a persuasion–resistance trap: The harder you persuade, the more the patient resists. A good guide never gets too far out in front.

PRACTITIONER: [feeling great concern for the patient] Unless you quit using drugs, you are going to lose your child. Have you thought about some treatment that might help with this?

PATIENT: My problem is the money, like I take these men in [prostitution] to feed me and my baby, and the heroin helps me to survive.

RESCUING THE PATIENT

Another common response to strong feelings of wanting patients to change is to try to rescue them. This can take many forms, from excessive enthusiasm, urging, and pleading to offering lots of support or even breaking role and visiting them at home to putting your hand into your pocket to offer money, and so on. Perversely, rescuing can sometimes be the last thing the person needs, because you might be unwittingly reinforcing his or her role as a victim awaiting your solution. Kindness can be taken too far, particularly when it substitutes for actions that patients themselves could take.

JUST FOLLOWING THE PATIENT AND GETTING LOST

If someone is struggling with bad news or loss, your heart goes out to him or her, and you know that just being with him or her and following his or her struggles can be quite helpful. A similar pattern can unfold in the discussion of behavior change, when your strong desire to help leads you to just listen (follow), and you lose control over the direction of the discussion. In some settings, in which you develop a relationship with the patient over numerous meetings, this pattern can go on for months or even years. If behavior change is one of the key issues facing the person, it can be productive to regain a little control over the direction of the discussion, perhaps by asking a guiding question or two, without losing your good relationship with the patient. Agenda setting can be a productive way of helping both of you stand back from the situation and consider options for behavior change. Being frank about this with the patient can also help.

OVERLOADING PATIENTS WITH INFORMATION

You feel very concerned; perhaps you don't have a lot of time, so you simply launch into providing information. There is a problem, you are the professional, you right the things that go wrong, and information transfer is in your toolbox. Combine this with a strong desire for the patient to change, and this tool can come out of the box in a flood of information that soon loses the attention of the passive patient.

PURSUING PROBLEMS AND WEAKNESSES

You sometimes feel so strongly about getting the job done and about where you feel the problem lies that you forget the patient's view and focus on the troubled zone of problem behavior with a determination that flattens the patient into defensiveness. Policing "bad" behavior replaces the opportunity to elicit the patient's strengths and aspirations.

Your positive aspirations for change in the patient can be a reflection of considered judgment and genuine concern, or they can be externally driven by guidelines and service protocols. The former can be used to good effect; the latter perhaps requires greater watchfulness on your part. Our aim here is not to turn you into a budding psychotherapist but simply to encourage you to be mindful of your own emotional reactions and how they can derail the guiding process.

Behavior-change consultations contain a mixture of your aspirations and those of the patient. How you steer a constructive path through this challenge is the next topic.

The Relationship: When Agendas Differ

Consider how a consultation might proceed under the circumstances presented in the simple two-by-two diagram in Figure 9.1. The most difficult scenarios are those in which there is a mismatch of aspirations (labeled with a danger sign in the figure).

When there is a mismatch between you and the patient—most commonly when your ABCs are high and the patient's aspirations are low—time can be wasted if you proceed as if the mismatch does not or should not exist. You might even feel that you are quietly trying to get around

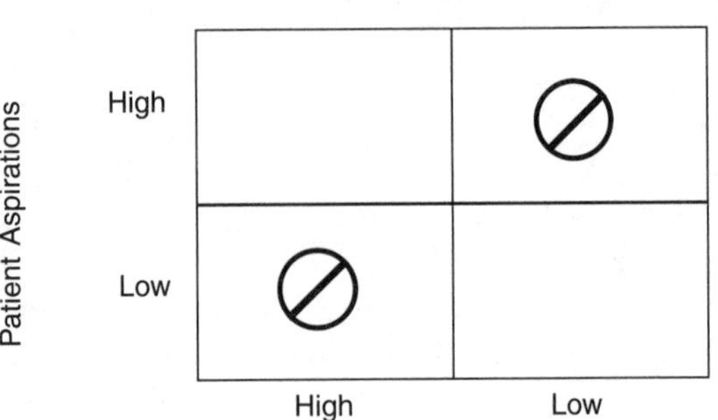

FIGURE 9.1. Aspirations for behavior change.

this mismatch, effectively nudging or even manipulating the patient this way and that. The empathy with and acceptance of the patient that lie at the heart of MI are soon undermined. In this situation, taking stock with the patient might help, and agenda setting is designed to do just this. A similar approach is also called for in the reverse situation, where patient aspirations are high and yours are low. For example, a patient very much wants a referral for surgery, while you are not at all convinced about this. At some point you might need to have an open discussion about this.

Agenda Setting

Agenda setting, introduced in Chapter 4, is a routine strategy for developing a compromise between your aspirations and agenda and those of the patient. The more you feel the need to impose your aspirations on the patient, the greater the need for clear agenda setting of this kind.

> "I want her to get more exercise and prepare for a return to work; she wants yet another note from me excusing her from work."
>
> "I want to focus on smoking, and he seems to think that a change in medication will solve everything."
>
> "Now he wants yet another referral for a scan, and he knows that I want him to look at the pressures in everyday life that probably cause these headaches."
>
> "She wants more and more pain killers, and I want to her to be more active."

Good rapport is invaluable in resolving these difficulties. In Chapter 4 we described a structured process of laying out all the possible topics one might talk about, providing both you and the patient the opportunity at the outset to agree on the way ahead. However, one can turn to a less structured form of agenda setting in the middle of a consultation in order to tackle a divergence in aspirations between you and the patient. For example, in the fourth scenario just described, in which the patient wants more pain killers and you feel that exercise might be better, you might do the following:

> *The more you feel the need to impose your aspirations on the patient, the greater the need for clear agenda setting.*

- Summarize how the patient is feeling and your understanding of her aspirations. This enhances rapport and ensures that the patient does not feel that you have misunderstood or are ignoring her needs.

- Proceed with agenda setting; for example:

  "Let's just take a step back for a minute and look at our progress. We both want you free of pain, that's for sure, and we can talk about different ways of getting there. There's taking more pain killers, something you want and that I have some concerns about, and then there's getting more exercise, which I favor and you have concerns about! So where do we go from here? Have I missed something?"

It is not advisable to be prescriptive about where you might go next in a difficult consultation such as this. However, agenda setting does give you more freedom, for example, to talk about your concerns about pain killers, particularly if you ask permission first. Conveying concern about the patient's well-being and using agenda setting to be open about different aspirations often leads to a more productive route through the impasse.

Tougher Consultations: Where Directing Seems Essential

Everyday practice yields pressures and predicaments that can confuse both you and your patient. You might ideally want to adopt a guiding style, but you have other roles as well, often defined by the service you work in. This can mean that you must at times depart from guiding and impose certain topics on the patient. Here are some examples.

- You want to help a troubled mother with behavior change because she might benefit from more social contact with others, from drinking less alcohol, and from new approaches to the behavioral problems of her children; but it is also your duty to consider the welfare of the children if they are at risk.
- Your service requires you to raise the subject of lifestyle change in a way that is not easy to integrate with a guiding style. There is a routine assessment that *must* be done.
- You feel obliged to warn a patient that a test result has some very clear implications for behavior change.
- A patient is in the habit of driving to the clinic intoxicated and is clearly a danger to others.

You might ideally want to adopt a guiding style, but you have other roles as well, often defined by the service you work in. This can mean that you must at times depart from guiding and impose certain topics on the patient.

If your service, role, or clinical judgment obliges you to adopt a directing style and impose a discussion of difficult topics on the patient, how might this obligation be integrated with a guiding style to be used for addressing behavior change? Here are some guidelines you might find useful, using the first example of the troubled mother.

- Put extra work into rapport building and listening, as close as possible to the beginning of the consultation.
- Clarify the challenge for both of you as soon as possible, ideally at the beginning of the consultation. You or your patients might find the metaphor of switching hats useful. Consider this approach:

> "A very important part of my job is to help you, in whatever way seems right for you. And I'd like to spend some time on this today [the guiding hat]. Then there's another part of my job [the directing hat] that means I must think about what's best for the children. So I switch between these two jobs. But I'd like to start with how I might be able to help you, because I know that a happier mother means happier children, if you see what I mean."

- If the problem arises in the middle of a consultation, take a break. Summarize where you are, step back with the patient, and address this problem. Try to be clear and honest, making sure that conveying respect for the patient is a high priority.
- If possible, start with the patient's concerns, and use a guiding style. Work hard on expressing acceptance and on demonstrating, with reflective listening, that you understand the patient's predicament, even if this is done briefly in just a few reflective listening statements.
- Make the changing of roles between guide and director explicit. This is what we mean by "changing hats." Try not to fudge or blur the distinction between these roles by winding your way through the conversation in a manner that might confuse the patient. For example, you might say:

> "I've talked about my different jobs, and we have spent quite a lot of time on how you might manage the kids better and get out of the house more, for your own sanity. Now I'd like to switch hats and talk only about the children, because I do have some concerns I'd like to ask you about. Is that OK?"

Make the changing of roles between guide and director explicit. This is what we mean by "changing hats." Try not to fudge or blur the distinction between these roles by winding your way through the conversation in a manner that might confuse the patient.

YOUR OWN HEALTH

Feeling responsible for changing the behavior of others can be wearing. As you get better at the guiding style of MI, you may find that this source of stress diminishes and that you learn to care for and about the patient without necessarily taking on the heavy burden of making behavior change happen.

With some release from feeling responsible come other challenges of a completely different kind: Your good work can take you close to the heart of the suffering associated with a patient's efforts to consider change. This, too, can take its toll on your well-being. Guiding is a delicate balance between coming close enough to your patients to understand and empathize with their experiences and retaining your separate role as a healer. In the biblical story, Moses finds his calling in life when his attention is captured by a bush that is burning and yet is not consumed. That is the healing balance: to burn without being consumed. A very experienced pediatrician once put it this way:

Guiding is a delicate balance between coming close enough to your patients to understand and empathize with their experiences and retaining your separate role as a healer.

> "Every family that comes to my attention has a story, and every story is interesting, and every story is different. I am never going to get burned out because I am interested in their stories. It's when I start to treat patients by checklists and formulas that I get bored, and that's when I am at risk for burnout."

LOOKING INTO YOUR OWN CONSULTATIONS

Something else that may help you to get better at guiding is to listen to recordings (made with patient permission, of course) of your own consultations. It is like an athlete watching a video of his or her own performance. You can observe more clearly where things went right and where they went wrong.

> "At first, it felt like I was handing all control over to them, and that there was no way I could even control the time, let alone get through what I wanted and needed to do. Then when I was listening to the recording of a consultation, I noticed this one open question that I asked. I was in control, but the patient was still moving. The consul-

tation had completely changed. I never knew at the time quite what had happened."

PRACTICING YOUR SKILLS IN EVERYDAY LIFE

There is a body of literature on mother–infant interaction that suggests that guiding is an apparently universal and natural communication style for helping infants to gain mastery over their new environment. *Scaffolding* or *guided participation* are terms used to describe how a good parent or tutor naturally structures a conversation so that the needs and abilities of the child are carefully addressed. The skillful parent or tutor does neither too much for the child (direct) nor too little, leaving the child to flounder (follow). Skillful guiding produces better learning outcomes.

Opportunities to practice guiding may include a conversation with a friend talking about a difficult decision. The temptation to leap in with solutions using a directing style is often strong. Listening, asking, suggesting, supporting, and encouraging are probably more useful and effective. Toward the end of life, elderly people frequently need to discuss difficult problems. What combination of listening, asking, and informing does one use? There is no formula here, but using these skills in the service of guiding is often more effective than simply directing them about how to resolve matters.

Listening can be practiced in almost any conversation, not only in the service of guiding. The first thing you may notice when trying to use reflections in everyday life is that attending to the wording of your reflection can take your focus away from a genuine interest in what the other person is saying. It is that initially clumsy feeling as you acquire skillfulness, but don't let it deter you. Keep going, because quite soon it should feel less contrived, and the reward will be there for you to reap.

> *Listening can be practiced in almost any conversation, not only in the service of guiding.*

Beneath all this focus on your skills lies something more important that extends beyond the technical. Through skillful listening and guiding, you are conveying a message of acceptance, hope, and compassion. This cannot be conjured up in an artificial way. In one sense, compassion, acceptance, and hope are your own internal experiences, but they are not of much use to patients until you communicate them. You can voice these things directly, of course: "I care"; "I think everything is going to be fine." Yet there is something particularly powerful about a compassionate, listening, guiding style that communicates hope and acceptance not just in what you say but in how you are with your patients. Chances are that the desire to be a healing presence for others is one of the reasons you chose your profession. The skills of reflective listening and the accompanying guiding are among the best ways to communicate your caring and acceptance. Practicing them also builds your capacity for acceptance and compassion.

CONCLUSION

This chapter concludes the account of the method of MI and how it can be used in some quite difficult circumstances in everyday health care. The next and final chapter turns to the application of MI in the wider clinical environment in which a service is delivered.

CHAPTER 10

Beyond the Consultation

The primary purpose of this book is to define and describe an approach to one-to-one health care consultations. We have encouraged you to use consultations to help patients explore their own ambivalence about change and to maximize their control over their own health. In this chapter we offer some examples in which MI was afforded a happy marriage with the system within which it was used. We hope they show how MI can be successfully integrated into services that meet the needs of patients and also promote behavior change.

Individual consultations clearly have their limits. Forces outside of the consultation, in the clinic and beyond, pose obstacles to patient change. Economic and social conditions often hold sway over people's efforts to improve their health and lifestyles. Forces within the service also affect your work. For example, if the service or health care system reinforces patient passivity, your best efforts to promote change through individual consultations can be undermined.

> "Next, please [after a 1-hour wait in a full waiting room]. Thank you, Ms. Evans. Can I ask you to please get undressed to your underwear and put this gown on? I'll come back and do your vital signs, OK? Then you'll see the nurse and then. . . ."

If you have a consultation about behavior change after the patient has been subjected to this kind of routine, it will be that much harder to accomplish guiding successfully, with its emphasis on the patient who is actively considering options and taking charge of changes in his or her life. Moreover, if many of your colleagues are not committed to adopting a more collaborative approach to their communication with patients, you might well wonder about the impact of your individual work.

These barriers within the health care system and beyond will influence your patients' motivations for health change behavior. *Can a health care system be changed so that barriers are removed and practitioners are better able to integrate a guiding style into their everyday practice?* Our starting point here is that we can and should be doing these things. Our goal is to identify signposts of change in health service delivery. We do this fully aware that this challenge of changing systems has been addressed by others with experience and knowledge far greater than ours. However, thoughtful changes in a health care practice or system can make a big difference in what happens in the consulting room and can make a guiding style easier to use and more effective.

The accounts that follow come from actual clinical practice settings. We have spoken to the practitioners involved at some length and have come to know them and their services quite well. The descriptions and quotations are accurate in spirit but have been adjusted to preserve anonymity where appropriate. The first set of examples focuses on removing general system obstacles; the second set involves efforts directly to use MI in health care.

REMOVING BARRIERS TO CHANGE

In these two examples, system changes helped to make the service more accessible to patients and their needs and encouraged them to make choices about behavior change whenever possible. Before the changes, it seemed all but impossible to integrate MI into the system. Afterward, it became something that the staff was eager to embrace.

1. Redesigning a Service

Setting and problem: Outpatient clinic for detoxification and treatment of substance abuse.

Goals: To improve attendance; to engage patients more actively in treatment; to promote change in substance use.

Before

The program staff members were competent and well intentioned but also discouraged and demoralized. Every day they saw people whose lives had been devastated and who were dependent on alcohol and other drugs of abuse. The medical staff provided high-quality outpatient detoxification services, after which substance abuse treatment was available on site. Yet many patients failed to keep their appointments, even for initial evaluation. Many who did complete the evaluation and detoxification never returned for ongoing treatment. Some of them would appear again months later, once again acutely ill. There was a general attitude of pessimism and helplessness among the staff that these patients were generally ungrateful, rude, resistant, unmotivated, and in denial. Staff turnover was high, as was absenteeism. Quarrels among different members of the team were common.

Now look for a moment through the eyes of a patient trying to get help through this service. Appointments could not be made over the telephone. Rather, patients, most of whom were poor, had to report by 8:00 A.M., when the intake window opened. The clinic itself was located in a warehouse district some distance from the nearest transportation line, and it could be a 2-hour journey to reach the clinic via public transport. The intake window was literally that: a small glass window in a wall behind which the staff worked. The window opened onto a hallway that was rather dark and often cold in wintertime. There were four or five old chairs in the hallway, and other patients had to stand. The normal morning traffic passed by them: staff members arriving for work, patients coming in for daily methadone, police and security personnel. By the time the window opened at 8:00, there was usually a line of people waiting. Because of the complexity of the intake process, only five or six could be seen. The rest were told to wait until the afternoon or to go home and try again the next day. The atmosphere at the intake window was often surly and chaotic.

Those who stayed were taken, one at a time, back into the medical clinic area. Some waited 2 hours before being taken inside. They first saw a nurse, who took vital signs and screened for acute detoxification needs. Next they spent about half an hour with a case worker, who determined their employment status, examined income verification (such as a paycheck stub), and asked a series of questions to determine eligibility for insurance or public support. If they were not screened out at this step, they next met with a different intake worker to complete a series of forms and a structured interview that asked a series of highly personal questions.

After this, they were given an appointment to return for the orientation, or "O," group, one of two weekly groups intended to prepare people for treatment. It also served as a holding system until patients could be assigned to a counselor, as well as a screen for "motivation." The O group was presented with a series of lectures and films about the harms of substance abuse, and patients on average attended 4–6 sessions before being assigned to a counselor. Then they would be given the name of their counselor and an appointment time to return to begin treatment. Only a small fraction of patients who appeared at the intake window made it all the way to a first counseling appointment. For those who did, the treatment they received was whatever the counselor deemed appropriate.

System Changes

New management offered some new resources and the opportunity to create changes in this service delivery system. The goal was to create a clinic that was welcoming and accessible and that delivered effective services as quickly and to as many patients as possible. A set of "seven C's" was developed as guiding principles for this new patient-centered model of care:

1. *Courtesy*: Every patient, caller, and colleague is treated in a courteous and respectful manner every time.
2. *Collaboration*: Staff members have a sense of common purpose and cooperation toward shared goals. Most goals are met through collaborative rather than solo efforts.
3. *Contribution*: Every person carries a fair share of the work to be done, looking for ways to make personal contributions to common mission and goals.
4. *Conscientiousness*: Every person is committed to promoting excellence of services and is conscientious with regard to work schedules and standards.
5. *Communication*: There is open communication throughout the clinic. Concerns are raised and information is checked directly with those involved.
6. *Connection*: Members of each unit understand their connection to the whole organization and are committed to the common vision and mission of the clinic.
7. *Community*: Every person shares a sense of common responsibility for the atmosphere, appearance, and services of the clinic and for the welfare of all patients.

Many practical changes were made over the course of a year. The intake window wall was torn down, creating a comfortably lighted and heated waiting area with ample seating, separated from the entry hallway. Patients were welcomed and offered coffee on arrival. Both walk-in and appointment options were available throughout the day. A patient feedback box was installed, with encouragement to comment both on problems and on good service received. The intake system was streamlined. Much of the essential information was collected via a questionnaire completed in the waiting room, with help available for patients who had difficulty reading or understanding it. The first person they saw was not a caseworker asking them questions but an experienced senior counselor who said, "I will need to ask you a few questions after a while, but right now I just want to hear what brings you in today. Tell me what's happening." A half hour of high-quality listening followed, which usually provided most of the specific information needed. The goal was to enhance motivation for change and to provide a service that would likely be helpful even if this were the patient's only visit.

The clinic also developed a menu of different evidence-based group and individual treatment options, which were available at various times of the day or evening. Hours of service were extended without increasing overall staffing. The orientation group was discontinued, and instead patients were given, at intake, a list and explanation of the services available and were helped to choose from the menu the services they wanted and needed. Every effort was made to get each patient connected with a counselor and started in treatment within 1 week. Often the patient was able to meet his or her counselor during the intake or detoxification process.

The impact on both patients and staff was remarkable. Patient retention increased dramatically, and, after some turnover of staff members who preferred the old system, so did staff retention. Instead of blaming patients for being unmotivated, staff members came to see ambivalence as normal and thought of tackling low motivation as part of their job. The clinic survived through a managed-care era in which many others closed, and a comprehensive follow-up evaluation showed excellent patient outcomes comparable to those seen in well-controlled clinical trials.

A sense of shared common values runs through the heart of this story, even though the initial impetus for change came about in a top-down manner, with a shift in management. The latter is not essential for redesigning the service. We have encountered a service for adolescents with diabetes in which a team of practitioners decided to take a new approach to the problem of poor attendance and low levels of glycemic control among their patients. The patients were asked what they would prefer, and the clinic's hours of service were shifted to late afternoon to give them time to arrive from school and college. Then a subtler shift began to take place. The clinic staff moved from a "weight and bloods" service to something more relaxed, thoughtful, and attuned to patient needs. This quiet transformation ended up in something very different from the starting point: a service in which the young people walked in and were asked, "Who would you like to see first today?" The atmosphere, the conduct of consultations, and the selection of treatment options followed a very similar pattern to those just described in the substance abuse clinic. Attendance improved. The team started with shared values and a single innovation. This next example illustrates further how following this principle can bear fruit.

2. A Single Innovation

The following example, which we have tracked for a number of years, comes from the developing world. The team, working in one of the largest teaching hospitals in Africa, was faced with a desperate situation: poor adherence to treatment for a life-threatening condition among poverty-stricken patients.

Setting and problem: Inpatient and outpatient service for children with HIV/AIDS; poor adherence to treatment.

Goals: To promote adherence to antiretroviral therapy; to improve economic and social integration of mothers; to change the program to encourage healthier lifestyles in patients.

Before

More than 150 mothers were registered with the service, and they needed to give their children a regular regimen of medication for a life-threatening condition. The team could not stress the importance of adherence highly enough; good timing was essential, each day. The rates were low, and it was demoralizing for all concerned. The referral rates were rising. The mothers and their children had HIV/AIDS.

A typical journey for the mothers started in the acute pediatric admission ward. If the baby or child survived an acute infection, he or she was transferred to outpatient care. Then the trouble began. Attendance at subsequent appointments was sporadic, and it seemed difficult to "get through to" the mothers about the importance of adherence. They had a bewildered look about them. Communication difficulties abounded, and staff members regarded many mothers as being "in denial." Very few had jobs; they mostly lived in grossly substandard housing; and they found it very difficult to afford transportation to attend their routine outpatient appointments. In their culture, HIV was a source of shame. If they did take Western medicines, many stopped when they or their children seemed better, leading to multiple medical and public health problems. "When the mothers get angry," one nurse remarked, "we know we are starting to make progress. It means there is hope." Mostly, however, passivity was the norm. Antiretroviral therapy had recently become available, but how could adherence be improved?

System Changes

The change in service design and delivery can be described quite well by following the journey of a new mother. She is literally penniless and lives with 12 others in a shack in a large township. She is brought by ambulance to the hospital with her very sick child. She spends most of the next fortnight on the ward, and the child starts to recover from a serious acute respiratory infection. Soon after arrival, the mother is taken down the corridor to the outpatient waiting area, where she is introduced to one of the counselors, who gives her a cup of coffee and a sandwich. She meets other mothers, who sit around a table. This waiting area is alive with the atmosphere of a small market. Mothers are making beadwork. A candle is placed in the middle of the table for cutting the nylon thread they use. The new mother learns about how she can get work. She starts to talk with others about the life she leads. Children are playing on and around the floor, taking turns being seen by a doctor to monitor their condition and the use of antiretroviral medicine. They seem mostly quite well.

When the child is discharged from inpatient care, the mother is given an outpatient appointment and a single bag of beads and some thread, having been taught to make strings for conference badge holders by another mother. She returns the next week. She and her child are seen by a doctor. On either side of this consultation, she meets more mothers, and the best of her beadwork is bought from her at the nurse's duty desk, to be sold by a small charity.

Over the next few months, she learns from other mothers about antiretroviral medication use. She forms friendships and talks about the difficult issue of HIV status disclosure. She also has the opportunity to talk informally or privately with any of the counselors working in the clinic, many of whom are HIV-positive themselves and have volunteered to help others. She uses the income from her first bag of beads to buy more, and she now has full-time work and makes regular return visits to the clinic, where they have set up a bank account for her.

"Just imagine," said the lead pediatrician, "the lives these patients lead. It's really impossible to imagine. I try, but I cannot." Looking back, the change process emerged from an experience of profound empathy. Glimpses into their lives prompted action.

"We were treating only one part of the problem," he remarked some years later. "If people don't have adequate food in their stomachs, it impacts on our treatment, and if we do nothing about this, the medical problems return to haunt us. The point is this: Our responsibilities can and should go beyond the treatment of the individual. We decided to develop a socioeconomic intervention within the walls of our hospital."

What started as an apparently narrow innovation designed to provide work and money for transportation now helps to break down other barriers: social isolation, difficulty with status disclosure, understanding how medication works, and overcoming a wide range of personal and social obstacles. Treatment for the children, if they adhere to their medication regimens, is starting to look like the management of other chronic illnesses such as diabetes, rather than like terminal care. This model of good practice is being replicated elsewhere (see *www.kidzpositive.org*). The staff members have now received initial training in MI, which is entirely congruent with the ethos of the service and the emphasis on patient empowerment. The counselors are developing a professional identity, they meet with the pediatrician each week, and they also network with other teams treating children in other African countries (*www.teampata.org*).

This kind of innovation is not unique. Simply moving a clinic from a hospital into the community can make a big difference. Indeed, the growth of primary care across the world could be seen as an effort to improve access and continuity of care that makes a real impact on people's lives. Numerous examples of community initiatives in health and social care illustrate the value of reaching out to improve awareness, to educate people about important issues, to provide better care, and even to improve their economic circumstances. Health behavior change is more likely to occur under these circumstances.

IMPLEMENTING MI

In the preceding examples, the use of MI emerged as a by-product of more fundamental service improvement. In this section, attention turns to direct efforts to introduce MI into a system. In the first example, training in MI led to complementary changes in service delivery. In the second, MI was used as the framework for health promotion in a water purification program in a developing country.

Training in MI and Other Changes

Setting and problem: Inpatient and outpatient hospital service; cardiac rehabilitation.

Goals: To change the program to encourage healthier lifestyles in patients; to encourage staff to learn MI; to adjust routines and procedures in line with a guiding style.

This brief account describes work in progress, which should afford you the opportunity to get a better feel for the unfolding nature of change within a system and for the challenges involved. It could be of interest to virtually any team working within primary or secondary care.

Before

By the time the patients had passed through their immediate crises, they seemed passive, frightened, and sometimes depressed, whether they had undergone surgery or not. They were used to being told of the need to get more exercise, to control their diets, to stop smoking, and so on. If they had had problems before they came into the hospital, they now had quite a few more to contend with. They came from diverse cultural backgrounds. On discharge, they were invited back into the cardiac rehabilitation service as outpatients. Attendance was reasonable, but many dropped out before completing the program.

Staff morale was low, primarily as a result of feeling the pressure of working with a high caseload and of feeling that it was their responsibility to *make* patients change their behavior. The team, comprising many nurses, a psychologist, a physiotherapist, and a dietician, offered a multiphased rehabilitation program, which began with an assessment and included such components as educational group meetings, relaxation training, and individual consultations. The emphasis was on helping people with long-term conditions to learn to make healthier choices of many kinds, much of the latter being lifestyle changes. Practitioners were clearly united by values that centered on helping patients to maximize opportunities for improving their health. The urgency of the need for changes in the patients' lifestyles confronted all involved. Education, education, education seemed to be the modus operandi of the service. Resistance, denial, and stubbornness were qualities frequently attributed to their patients. Could a shift in the way they talked with patients about change improve matters?

After

The team leader, a psychologist, showed an article on MI to a lead nurse, and they agreed that they were spending too much time deciding patient's priorities for them, giving advice and providing them with education of all kinds. Perhaps the attendance rates might improve if the team was offered the opportunity to learn a different approach. They organized a 2-day workshop on MI. They knew the direction they wanted to go in but were able to tolerate uncertainty about the pace and outcome of the change process. The team had never met together before outside of conventional case management meetings.

They closed the service for 2 days. Fourteen practitioners turned up at a country house, the training venue. They were soon engaged in pretraining simulated consultations, with actors playing roles of typical patients. Most had never heard about MI, and moving in and out of simulated exercises was also new to them. Struggles with shifting styles between directing and guiding were well matched by difficulties in actually formulating listening statements rather than asking questions. Handing over elements of responsibility for decisions to the patient seemed to be a major underlying challenge.

Then reality struck. The pace of routine clinical practice left many with no apparent alternative to the standard educational approach of advising patients why and how they should change. Putting MI skills into practice was clearly quite a challenge. It was not easy to remember what they had learned in the workshop. With no others around to observe their practice, or at least to discuss this with them, breaking old habits was not easy. Yet some had clearly made progress. One said, "I know sometimes I am talking with a patient and I think 'Ooooh—that was MI!' and I'm thinking I should do that more often. I try to be more conscious about using it." Another reported that the coronary care staff (not part of their team) saw him with patients and asked why he was not yelling at them about their smoking and telling them to stop eating junk food. He suggested that maybe these patients got tired of people standing at the end of their beds telling them that they will die if they do not do this and do that. One nurse summed it up along these lines: "You know when you've got it right because you get a nice buzz back from the patient, and you know when you've got it horribly wrong because you get a negative response—it's the in-between that's tricky; you're missing subtleties, aren't you?"

Discussion in the coffee room about further learning included suggestions about shorter booster workshops, peer-support meetings, reading transcripts, listening to audio recordings, sitting in on each other's consultations, and scoring one's own consultation using a checklist. Yet the senior practitioners who had initiated the workshops and had participated with enthusiasm were not inclined to follow these ideas. They had a larger idea: culture change, to examine together the way in which the service routines reinforced or undermined behavior change.

TEAM MEETINGS

The team was offered a series of 2-hour "team meetings" to consider how the service might be adjusted in line with the principles of a guiding rather than a directing style. Initially, the facilitator tried to elicit from the members what changes they would like to make, after which their attention focused on two topics, assessment and groups. They had five meetings in all, spread out over a period of 3 months, and all involved agreed that it got better as they went along. To begin with, they said, things seemed a little unfocused. As they got better at working together and reaching agreement about changes to the service, their everyday practice became more innovative and mutually supportive. The term *culture change* was widely used in their discussions, and they seemed better able to tolerate individual and professional differences. "Now," said one practitioner, "I get e-mails and telephone calls from others in the team asking for help with problems."

CHANGING ASSESSMENT PROCEDURES

The first meeting with a new patient involved a lengthy assessment that took, on average, 30 minutes. The typical pattern was for the practitioner to use a directing style to elicit answers to a sequence of set questions and to fill this information in as they went along. Initial efforts to make the changes agreed on in the team meetings were frustrating, because the practitioners felt that the forms still dictated the course of the conversation and that the patients merely responded to this process. They wanted the assessment to have a less "clinical" feel, to be more of a two-way process, one in which the patient was also given the chance to consider his or her aspirations for behavior change.

They made more substantial changes to the order of questions. They inserted some new ones that elicited the patient's views about the origins of their heart disease and about their beliefs and aspirations for lifestyle change. Some questions of a factual nature were left to the end. The assumption was that if the patient was active in the assessment process, answers to these questions would probably emerge in the natural course of the conversation. A new "crib sheet" was constructed so that the discussion could flow freely from the patient's perspective, with the practitioner making sure that all the topics were being covered. Then the form was completed.

The assessment process clearly became more interesting for both parties. One practitioner commented, "I'm astounded at the stories I get told by people who maybe have had angina for 20 years, but their understanding of it is really bizarre sometimes." Another noted:

> "I find the new bits of the assessment very useful because asking the patient what they think happened to them and what brought them here is just such a useful tool. There was no space for that in the previous form. And also things like asking them what their primary concern is, which is often not their cardiac condition, but their heart

> attack is meaningless against the fact that their wife is really ill, or children taking drugs, and it does put it into context—they will come to our service but they may not find it as interesting as you expect them to. I find that really useful."

Getting a feel for the whole person, including his or her views about where lifestyle change might fit in, made it easier to decide what to focus on in later consultations. Some claimed that this assessment took longer than the old procedure; others disagreed and teased their colleagues for being "slow coaches."

PATIENT EDUCATION GROUPS

The team ran a sequence of educational topic-driven "talks" each week. They decided to rely less on PowerPoint presentations, they changed the order of topics, and they constructed guidelines for handling questions and observations from patients. The most radical change was a newly constructed final session with an open-ended format to explore struggles with behavior change, following the principles of MI.

The groups provided practitioners with their one opportunity to actually work together in pairs. One of the problems with a less structured format was letting go of the well-intentioned impulse to provide patients with every bit of information they felt they needed. The payoff was greater involvement from the patients.

> "It's difficult. It's more difficult because I'm so used to just giving the information and that's it, and then you ask questions at the end, but this is almost like open forum and you know what—I think they get more from it. . . . More people start throwing in their ideas, then somebody else will and somebody else. The person you would least expect to say something just comes out and says something and you think, fantastic. . . . And they seem more enthusiastic about things then. Instead of just standing up there and giving them the information we're now looking at the patients' needs and what they need is not always what you imagine . . . so I think I've become more sympathetic toward patients that way, emotionally. Definitely."

Over the first few months, the team learned about the circumstances in which particular questions were useful in group discussions. Asking about importance and confidence (see Chapter 4) was apparently very helpful in talk about medication use. Use of a pros-and-cons strategy (Chapter 4) they found more generally applicable and especially useful in talk about exercise: "This is very good for finding gaps in their understanding, like it seems that 90% of the patients don't think of walking as exercise." On the subject of feedback, one nurse said, "Well, I think it's stopped us pussyfooting around the patients as well. You know, we allow patients to tell us what they think ought to be the feedback, and they allow us to tell them what we think ought to be in feedback, and I think we meet in the middle."

Changes in one part of the program affected others. One practitioner was heard to say, "After trying this out for the first time in groups, I have this sort of conversation outside of the group as well, so the one feeds into the other for me." This process affected even those who had not attended the initial MI training. "There are some members of the team who never came into the training, and they've learned from the way we are managing the groups, and they're changing what they do, which is really interesting."

In interviews a year later, staff members agreed that throwing everyone together in the same workshop on a subject they knew little about was a great leveler. It brought them together across professional boundaries with a legitimate focus. The use of practical exercises was not suited to everyone's taste or learning style. One nurse said, "I hated the groups (simulations), sitting around and dragging things out of people, but I loved the MI."

Commentary

With commitment and creativity, change in an organization or service is achievable and will enhance patient health behavior change. The process of gradual change mirrors the most frequent pattern of behavior change among patients. Attention is focused on both the *why* and the *how* of behavior change. In the preceding example, team meetings and training events served to highlight not just what to do—the *how* of change—but also the *why* of change—their commitment to shifting their service in line with more effective and respectful ways of promoting health behavior change. Tolerance of uncertainty and ambivalence, setting achievable goals, and reviewing progress are all individual-practitioner behavior-change issues that required mindfulness and a firm guiding style from team leaders themselves. Essentially, the whole team became better at guiding:

> "It's useful for me to talk to that person as an individual and find out what is important to them about becoming fitter. It might be something simple like being able to do the housework, or somebody else could be wanting to run a marathon, so it's good really to find out what that individual's needs are really and how far they want to go—

and how far they can go with other problems as well. So that has helped me as well to sort of relate to them as an individual."

The interest in using groups conducted along these lines of MI has grown considerably in recent years. Table 10.1 contains some general guidelines constructed with two colleagues who have worked on this topic in a number of settings.

MI and Public Health Promotion

In the developing world, access to safe drinking water is a major health problem, and diarrhea caused by water-borne organisms is a leading cause of death for children under the age of 5. Relatively simple and inexpensive water purification methods are available and effectively reduce disease and death from contaminated water supplies. The most common methods used to persuade families to adopt water purification methods are educational in nature, passing on "why" and "how" information. However, for a variety of reasons, such educational strategies can be ineffective in promoting this life-saving behavior change.

Such was the case in regions of Zambia. In an attempt to address this problem, Dr. Angelica Thevos and her colleagues tried a unique experiment. They identified two communities without water systems, in which utilization of chlorine for water purification remained low. Ten health promotion volunteers serving these areas were divided into two teams of five. The team serving one area received no additional training and continued to use the educational materials (fliers, flip-chart-guided talks) to introduce families to the chlorination procedures. The team serving the other area was given 5 hours of training in MI specifically adapted to the subject of water purification, including role-play practice exercises.

Over the next 8 months, the team used a simple, unobtrusive measure to evaluate the adoption of water purification: the number of bottles of sodium hypochloride sold in each locale. They reported a large effect ($p < .001$), with chlorine sales being two to four times higher in the community visited by MI-trained volunteers.* A single study seldom provides definitive answers. You might wonder, for example, what exactly the trained health promotion volunteers did in their conversations with people. However, both this example and that of the cardiac rehabilitation team strongly suggest that trainers, researchers, and practitioners

* Thevos, A. K., Quick, R. E., & Yanduli, V. (2000). Application of motivational interviewing to the adoption of water disinfection practices in Zambia. *Health Promotion International*, *15*(3), 207–214.

TABLE 10.1. Guidelines for Guiding in Groups

Principles

In addition to the fundamental principles of collaboration, evocation, and honoring autonomy (see Chapter 1), consider these additional possibilities that apply specifically to the group setting:

Avoid traps

- Don't conduct multiple individual consultations in a group setting.
- Avoid question and answer sessions conducted by you, the expert.
- Avoid allowing the group to become either too unfocused or too serious.

Golden rules

- Remember your goal: to bring everyone together to focus on a topic and gain support from one another.
- Link individual stories to topic and experience of others. Extract the essence of the patient's story and broaden it out. A skillful facilitator will reframe "interrupting" as redirecting.
- Encourage the quiet, soften the loud. For example, you might ask quiet members to summarize some part of the group discussion and discuss how it fits for them. You might ask talkative members to summarize their points and pose a question to the group.
- Minimize negative interactions. Participants can overdo giving advice to others or even confront their apparent "denial" or excuse for avoiding change. Don't let negative interactions escalate. Remain empathic and supportive, but act immediately to regain control when group processes are going in a negative direction. Ask participants to reframe their advice to others into statements of "what has worked for me."
- Keep the focus of the group on enhancing motivation to change, increasing hope, and reducing the sense of burden that change imposes. Don't allow the groups to become exploratory psychotherapy groups or complaint sessions.

Topics and strategies

- *Past successes*: Focusing on things that participants have achieved can help to restore self-confidence and spark creativity in regard to the current change.
- *Ambivalence*: Focusing on participants' mixed feelings about change can help reduce defensiveness while preparing them to both initiate change and prevent relapse.
- *Values*: Supporting participants in examining how their current behavior fits with their core values can enhance motivation to change and help them find an internal source of direction to rely on when the status quo is threatening to take the upper hand.
- *Looking forward*: Helping participants envision a better future, rather than falling into a pattern of begrudgingly acknowledging and exploring past failures, can positively affect the relationship between the participants and their struggles to change.
- *Exploring strengths*: Eliciting participants' sense of their own strengths can enhance their self-esteem and help them find internal resources that can support their current change effort. With mature groups, leaders can facilitate sharing of impressions of one another's strengths. This can be a quite powerful, supportive experience.
- *Planning change*: Using discussion and worksheets to plan change alone, in pairs, or as a large group can help transform vague motivation into concrete

(*continued*)

TABLE 10.1. (*continued*)

plans that help in initiating and maintaining change. Encourage participants to state one small change they are committing to rather than making a grand but vague plan. Follow up on how these commitments went in the next group meeting.

- *Exploring importance and confidence*: Using importance and confidence rulers to examine the relationship between participants and their change plans helps participants to see that these internal cognitive and emotional elements can either support them in their change efforts or hold them back.

Note. Written with Drs. Karen Ingersoll and Chris Wagner. Reprinted with permission from the authors.

themselves can explore, evaluate, and implement strategies that are based on the principles and practice of MI. A listing of research studies can be found in Appendix B.

CONCLUSION

The preceding examples illustrate various ways in which changes were made in service systems beyond the individual office consultation to promote patient well-being and health behavior change. A happy coincidence exists between the goals of patient empowerment initiatives such as those described in this chapter and the use of MI. The former makes the latter easier to use. Both need attention to succeed, and both involve practitioners who respond creatively to patient predicaments, who convey respect, hope, flexibility, and skill inside the consultation and beyond. It is one thing to sit with an individual patient and demonstrate restraint, tolerance of uncertainty, and trust in his or her ability to make good decisions; it is quite another to offer a service in which there is collective adherence to these values and skills.

In essence, we encourage you to try this collaborative, empathic guiding style in your individual practice and to think creatively about how health care delivery systems can be modified to be more consistent with this patient-empowering approach. In so many modern health problems, patient behavior change is a vital component of prevention and treatment. Practitioners have much control over prescriptions and procedures but little direct control when it comes to patients' behavior, in which a more collaborative approach is needed. MI is often effective in evoking behavior change when education and exhortation have failed. It is not every clinician's cup of tea, but if you like the flavor of it, you have a lifetime of practice ahead of you in which to try it out. We conclude the book with a brief, practical epilogue and two appendices with information about learning and research.

Epilogue

Some Maps to Guide You

LEARNING MI

Acquiring skill in MI is more complex and more satisfying than just learning a few new techniques. There is a more fundamental learning process in which you become comfortable with a shift to a guiding style, let go of the righting reflex, and instead trust the wisdom of your patients. Once you feel comfortable with this shift in approach when talking about health behavior change, more learning follows.

Oversimplifying a bit, we break the learning process down into three phases.

Phase 1: Shifting Styles with Comfort

Here you grasp the differences between styles (directing, guiding, and following), and how the three core skills (asking, listening, and informing) vary in both quality and quantity across them (Chapter 2). You notice what happens with your patients when you shift styles and develop the ability to do this comfortably and naturally. When you shift into guiding, try to retain control of the direction of the consultation, but leave it up to the patient to voice why and how he or she might change. This lifts from you the constant burden of being responsible for making change happen.

Practice verbally expressing the four RULE principles (Chapter 1) with patients during normal consultations. Choose your moment, shift to a guiding style, and let them know that you don't want to rush in and provide solutions (Resist the righting reflex), that you want to know how they really feel about change (Understand their motivations) by Listening, and that you believe that they can find solutions (Empower them). Consider using practical aids such as an agenda-setting chart or a readiness ruler to help you (Chapter 4) clarify what the patient wants to talk about and how ready he or she is to change. Use more open than closed questions (Chapter 4). Practitioners often find that they get quite different responses from patients when they shift into a guiding style, even early in the learning process. You can see the fruits of learning relatively soon, and sometimes consultations take on a dramatically different tone than they have before.

One other technique in this early phase is very useful: the summary (Chapter 5). When you make the shift to guiding, the patient usually becomes verbally more active, and quite a lot is said, often in just a minute or two. It can feel a little overwhelming. You might wonder whether you are losing control of both the time and the direction of the discussion. Offer a summary of what's been said. You'll find the patient appreciative and able to change direction if you so wish.

You know you are making progress when shifting back and forth between styles starts to feel less like a major event and more like an easy part of a normal conversation. This kind of experience can provide you with encouragement to learn more.

Phase 2: Getting Better at Guiding

Once you are comfortable with the value of a guiding style, you start becoming more skillful at it. You develop time-efficient ways of setting an agenda (Chapter 4). This usually ensures that the patient is "on board" and that good rapport is maintained. Formulate simple open questions about behavior change (Chapter 4) and use listening statements as a way of weaving your way through brief explorations of the why and how of change (Chapter 5). Practice using longer summaries to bring together what's been said, encourage progress, and shift direction as needed (Chapter 5). Through all of this, keep a sense of curiosity and patience, holding back your righting reflex more consistently. Again, a saving grace is that practitioners often see significant shifts in behavior-change consultations when they try out even a few of the skills, such as asking open questions, reflecting, and summarizing, in the course of daily practice.

Phase 3: Refining Your MI Skills

Once you get comfortable with the appropriate shift of a guiding style and how to use the basic core skills in this way, the rest is refinement. As described earlier, you learn to hear and attend to your patients' change talk, which tells you when you're doing it right. Your patients become your teachers. You find a range of open questions that work for you to open up conversations about behavior change and to elicit change talk. The simpler the better. You begin identifying the rich array of change talk in patients' speech. You notice what happens when you make a listening statement immediately afterward. Try reflecting different elements of patients' speech, particularly their change talk. Practice collecting change talk in longer summaries using the patient's own language, connected to his or her values and aspirations.

In the course of training and research, we have found that within the good practice of MI there is a wide range of personal approaches. The three of us, in fact, practice rather differently, yet we are manifesting the same underlying guiding style. It is in this third phase that you make MI your own, finding what works for you in helping your patients make health behavior changes.

A CONSULTATION GUIDE

No two consultations are alike, yet patterns often arise, for better or worse, usually highlighted by junctions that signal a shift in topic or perhaps in the style used by the practitioner. In a constructive consultation with a patient who has recently received bad news, for example, most practitioners would use a following style to begin with, and then ask whether the patient has any questions. Elements of a guideline for good practice can thus be constructed, as long as they contain flexibility that allows for the uniqueness of each consultation and the participants within it.

In the consultation about behavior change the most important element we have highlighted in this book is what we called the *spirit* of the conversation, where a guiding style is used to elicit from the patient their own good reasons for change.

Some practitioners report a sort of "freezing" experience, where all is going well, until they suddenly feel unsure about where to go next. The guideline that they simply adhere to the spirit of the method seems insufficient to help them through this kind of impasse. Might a more concrete guideline be helpful?

We've constructed one below, despite concerns about inadvertently promoting a formulaic approach to behavior change consulting. It's a deliberately rough guide, one that is best viewed as an adjunct to the basic need to keep to the spirit of the consultation emphasized in so many places in this book.

1. Agree on the Focus

Establish rapport. Fundamental to good practice is the simple notion that the more friendly and supportive the atmosphere, the more the patient feels understood by you, the better will be progress within and beyond the consultation.

Set agenda (Chapters 4 and 9). If there is only one behavior that is relevant (e.g., smoking), then this task is usually straightforward. You raise the subject and ask permission to talk about it. If there are a number of interrelated behaviors that could be addressed, invite the patient to consider the range of possibilities, paying attention to their preferences and readiness to change (Chapter 4), while being honest about your concerns. Reach agreement about a specific behavior on which to focus.

Emphasize the spirit of your approach to the consultation (Chapter 1). Simple messages can convey a great deal. They also help you to settle into a guiding style, and to make this clear to the patient. For example, a single sentence or two can convey quite a lot: "I see my job as not to lecture you about what you could change, but more as guide, using my experience with other patients to help you make decisions that make sense to you. I'd like to start by understanding what you really feel about change, is that OK?"

2. Explore and Build Motivation to Change

This is the heart of the discussion about behavior change, where you are listening for change talk, and inviting the patient to amplify why and how they might change. Among the possibilities open to you are:

Exchange information (Chapter 6). Using something like the elicit–provide–elicit framework can do much to enhance motivation to change.

Ask useful guiding questions (Chapter 4). Combine these with reflective listening (Chapter 5), effectively an invitation to clarify how the patient feels and to consider different perspectives, with a keen eye on the link between behavior change and their core values.

Consider using structured strategies (Chapter 4). For example, "Pros and Cons" and "Assessing Importance and Confidence" are designed to open the door to eliciting the patient's own motivation to change (change talk).

3. Summarize Progress

Among the possibilities here are:

Provide a long summary (Chapter 5). Follow this by asking the patient what the next step might be.

Return to agenda setting (Chapter 4). To clarify progress and agree on the way ahead.

Consider the next step. Clarify any plans for the future that you and the patient have agreed upon (e.g., follow-up visit, work on a specific and achievable goal).

APPENDIX A

Learning More about Motivational Interviewing

"Could you come and teach us motivational interviewing over the noon hour? A drug company is providing lunch." Such invitations are common, and they bespeak a misunderstanding of MI as a quick trick, a simple procedure that one could learn in a few minutes over pizza. Instead, think of MI as a complex clinical skill that is developed and refined over the course of one's career, much like learning to play chess or golf or the piano. A 1-hour lecture or even a full day of training is unlikely to engender much proficiency in such skills. The guiding style of MI is not a technique but a clinical method, a particular way of being with patients.

If MI is like chess, golf, or playing the piano, then one can expect at best modest gains from reading or hearing about it or even from watching videotape of the skilled practitioners. Practicing the fundamental shift to a guiding style can be done in everyday practice, in which the patient's reaction provides immediate opportunity for improving skill. Supporting this kind of learning in everyday practice is usually the best way to proceed.

It can be quite ambitious to expect practitioners to attend a workshop and return proficient in MI. We've tried. In one study, we randomized practitioners who wanted to learn MI to one of five training conditions. To one group we sent our book (Miller & Rollnick, 2002) and a set of training videotapes (Miller, Rollnick, & Moyers, 1998) and asked them to do their best to learn it on their own. Four months later, there was no improvement in performance (Miller, Yahne, Moyers, Martinez, & Pirritano, 2004). Skill improvement was also minimal in another group, who were given these resources and also received a 2-day clinical workshop with Dr. Miller (cf. Miller & Mount, 2001). Rather, proficiency in MI occurred only when one or both of two training aids were added: systematic feedback on performance and personal skill coaching. This makes sense, because feedback and expert coaching are precisely how one typically learns to master any complex skill. When we examined patient responses to the practitioners, the only group showing substantial improvement was the one that received both feedback and coaching, in addition to training (Miller et al., 2004).

By implication, we do not expect you to become proficient in MI just by reading this book nor even by going to an introductory lecture or workshop, though it can be a good start. You learn this method by doing it in a situation in which you can get feedback about how you're doing. Practice without feedback is not particularly helpful and can easily produce bad habits. It's rather like playing an electronic keyboard with the sound turned off. You can feel and imagine yourself performing the operations without the satisfaction (or dissatisfaction) of hearing the result.

AIDS TO LEARNING

One good aid to learning, then, is access to a clinician who is proficient in MI, someone who is more skillful at it than you are. You will also need to practice on your own, but short blocks of time with an expert coach can be very helpful. In order to help you, the coach will need to listen to your practice (perhaps by audiotape), much as a tennis coach needs to watch you and a piano teacher needs to hear you play. Many health care systems have done this by hiring a supervisor who is proficient in MI or bringing one of their current staff members up to such expertise through training. This person then can function as an in-house coach, helping other staff members to develop and strengthen their own clinical skills. This is quite different from a one-time training event in that the learning continues over time. Other systems and programs, lacking such an in-house expert, have set up ongoing peer consultations and support groups that meet regularly to discuss MI and listen to each other's practice.

Another option is to bring in an expert trainer once or periodically to help clinicians strengthen their practice. Repeated visits give clinicians the opportunity to try out learned skills in between training sessions and to bring questions and problems back to the trainer. One list of MI trainers is found at *www.motivationalinterview.org*, along with a description of training exercises often used to help practitioners learn this clinical method.

As discussed in many parts of this book, you also have at your disposal another very reliable source of performance feedback: your patients. Every time you practice MI, your patients give you clues as to how you are doing. Consider, for example, the component skill of reflective listening. Your patient discloses some personal information, and you do your best to respond with a reflective listening statement (Chapter 7). You get two immediate forms of feedback. First, the patient tells you whether or not the content of your reflection was correct:

PATIENT: I've been feeling kind of blue lately.

PRACTITIONER: You're feeling a little sad.

PATIENT: Yes, I can't really explain it, but I just break out crying over nothing.

Or

PATIENT: No, not sad really. It's more a lonely feeling.

Either way you get more information, and either way you're receiving feedback about the accuracy of your reflection. Second, if the patient keeps on talking to you, exploring the topic, and revealing more information, chances are you are doing it right.

Another important source of feedback is the patient's change talk (Chapter 5). At first you are asking and listening for DARN talk—desire, ability, reasons, and need for health behavior change. As you receive and collect these "flowers," you also reflect them and collect them in summary bouquets that you offer back to the patient. When you do this well, you begin hearing commitment language (Chapter 5), statements such as "I will" and "I am going to." These signal the kind of mental processing that leads, not always but usually, to behavior change.

Thus from your patients' own speech, what they say to you during consultations, you can get feedback about how you are doing in learning MI. It can be challenging at first to hear this in the midst of a consultation, and this is one reason that it can be helpful to tape-record some visits (with patient permission, of course) and review them later, either by yourself or with a consultant, trainer, or peer group. Trainers also sometimes review tapes by using a structured coding system that can yield a wealth of specific information. Several such systems have been published (Lane et al., 2005; Madson, Campbell, Barrett, Brondino, & Melchert, 2005; Miller & Mount, 2001; Moyers, Martin, Catley, Harris, & Ahluwalia, 2003; Moyers, Martin, Manuel, Hendrickson, & Miller, 2005; Rosengren, Baer, Hartzler, Dunn, & Wells, 2005).

The essential message here is that it takes time to develop skill in MI. One does not master it from reading or watching or from a single training. It can be slow going at first, as with any complex skill. Think of it as a learning process that happens over time, supported as feasible by feedback and coaching. It is a skill in which you can continue to improve for as long as you practice.

TRAINERS

For better or worse, we have made no attempt to restrict the practice or training of MI. There is currently no formal, accredited route to becoming a trainer of this clinical method. There is, however, an organization whose mission is to promote quality in the training of MI: the international Motivational Interviewing Network of Trainers (MINT). MINT operates an informational website (*www.motivationalinterview.org*) with a cumulative bibliography, extensive information about the clinical method, and a geographical listing of its members, who as of 2007 provide training in at least 27 languages. It also publishes a MINT Bulletin that is available online free of charge.

It is important to distinguish between teaching *about* MI (as one might do in a survey course) and providing clinical training in the method itself. Our perspective is that a competent trainer of MI should be quite proficient in delivering it. The MINT website includes an overview titled "What Might You Expect Out of Different Lengths and Types of Training?" that provides a good sense of the range of skills required of a trainer. There is also a manual containing a menu of exercises that MINT trainers use in various configurations.

If you are seeking a trainer, the MINT website is a good place to start. MINT periodically offers a 3-day specialized training for trainers that its own members have completed and that qualifies new trainers for membership in MINT. This does not in itself guarantee competence as a trainer, of course. If you are seeking a trainer or consultant, you might ask potential candidates about how much experience they have had working with practitioners in your area of expertise and for references from prior training events.

A BIBLIOGRAPHY ON TRAINING OF MI

Amrhein, P. C., Miller, W. R., Yahne, C., Knupsky, A., & Hochstein, D. (2004). Strength of client commitment language improves with therapist training in motivational interviewing. *Alcoholism: Clinical and Experimental Research*, *28*(5), 74A.

Baer, J. S., Rosengren, D. B., Dunn, C. W., Wells, W. A., Ogle, R. L., & Hartzler, B. (2004). An evaluation of workshop training in motivational interviewing for addiction and mental health clinicians. *Drug and Alcohol Dependence*, *73*(1), 99–106.

Bennett, G. A., Roberts, H. A., Vaughan, T. E., Gibbins, J. A., & Rouse, L. (2007). Evaluating a method of assessing competence in motivational interviewing: A study using simulated patients in the United Kingdom. *Addictive Behaviors*, *32*, 69–79.

Broers, S., Smets, E. M. A., Bindels, P., Evertsz, F. B., Calff, M., & DeHaes, H. (2005). Training general practitioners in behavior change counseling to improve asthma medication adherence. *Patient Education and Counseling*, *58*, 279–287.

Brug, J., Spikmans, F., Aarsen, C., Breedveld, B., Bes, R., & Ferreira, I. (2007). Training dietitians in basic motivational interviewing skills results in changes in their counseling style and in lower saturated fat intakes in their patients. *Journal of Nutrition Education and Behavior*, *39*(1), 8–12.

Burke, P. J., DaSilva, J. D., Vaughan, B. L., & Knight, J. R. (2006). Training high school counselors in the use of motivational interviewing to screen for substance abuse. *Substance Abuse*, *26*, 31–34.

Byrne, A., Watson, R., Butler, C., & Accoroni, A. (2006). Increasing the confidence of nursing staff to address the sexual health needs of people living with HIV: The use of motivational interviewing. *AIDS Care*, *18*, 501–504.

DeJonge, J. M., Schippers, G. M., & Schaap, C. P. D. R. (2005). The Motivational Interviewing Skill Code: Reliability and a critical appraisal. *Behavioural and Cognitive Psychotherapy*, *33*, 1–14.

Doherty, Y., Hall, D., James, P. T., Roberts, S. H., & Simpson, J. (2000). Change counselling in diabetes: The development of a training programme for the diabetes team. *Patient Education and Counseling*, *40*(3), 263–278.

Handmaker, N. S., Hester, R. K., & Delaney, H. D. (1999). Videotaped training in alcohol counseling for obstetric care practitioners: A randomized controlled trial. *Obstetrics and Gynecology*, *93*, 213–218.

Lane, C., Huws-Thomas, M., Hood, K., Rollnick, S., Edwards, K., & Robling, M. (2005). Measuring adaptations of motivational interviewing: The development and validation of the Behavior Change Counseling Index (BECCI). *Patient Education and Counseling*, *56*, 166–173.

Lane, C., Johnson, S., Rollnick, S., Edwards, K., & Lyons, M. (2003). Consulting about lifestyle change: Evaluation of a training course for specialist diabetes nurses. *Practical Diabetes International*, *20*, 204–208.

Levin, F. R., Owen, P., Stinchfield, R., Rabinowitz, E., & Pace, N. (1999). Use of standardized patients to evaluate the physicians in residence program: A substance abuse training approach. *Journal of Addictive Diseases*, *18*(2), 39–50.

Madson, M. B., & Campbell, T. C. (2006). Measures of fidelity in motivational enhancement: A systematic review. *Journal of Substance Abuse Treatment*, *31*, 67–73.

Madson, M. B., Campbell, T. C., Barrett, D. E., Brondino, M. J., & Melchert, T. P. (2005). Development of the Motivational Interviewing Supervision and Training Scale. *Psychology of Addictive Behaviors*, *19*, 303–310.

Miller, W. R., & Mount, K. A. (2001). A small study of training in motivational interviewing: Does one workshop change clinician and client behavior? *Behavioural and Cognitive Psychotherapy*, *29*, 457–471.

Miller, W. R., Moyers, T. B., Arciniega, L. T., Ernst, D., & Forcehimes, A. (2005). Training, supervision and quality monitoring of the COMBINE study behavioral interventions. *Journal of Studies on Alcohol* (Suppl. 15), 188–195.

Miller, W. R., & Rollnick, S. (2002). *Motivational interviewing: Preparing people for change* (2nd ed.). New York: Guilford Press.

Miller, W. R., Rollnick, S., & Moyers, T. B. (1998). *Motivational interviewing* [Videotape series]. Albuquerque: University of New Mexico.

Miller, W. R., Yahne, C. E., Moyers, T. B., Martinez, J., & Pirritano, M. (2004). A randomized trial of methods to help clinicians learn motivational interviewing. *Journal of Consulting and Clinical Psychology*, *72*, 1050–1062.

Mounsey, A. L., Bovbjerg, V., White, L., & Gazewood, J. (2006). Do students develop better motivational interviewing skills through role-play with standardized patients or student colleagues? *Medical Education*, *40*, 775–780.

Moyers, T. B., Martin, T., Catley, D., Harris, K. J., & Ahluwalia, J. S. (2003). Assessing the integrity of motivational interventions: Reliability of the motivational interviewing skills code. *Behavioural and Cognitive Psychotherapy*, *31*, 177–184.

Moyers, T. B., Martin, T., Manuel, J. K., Hendrickson, S. M. L., & Miller, W. R. (2005). Assessing competence in the use of motivational interviewing. *Journal of Substance Abuse Treatment*, *28*, 19–26.

Ockene, J. K., Wheeler, E. V., Adams, A., Hurley, T. G., & Hebert, J. (1997). Provider training for patient-centered alcohol counseling in a primary care setting. *Archives of Internal Medicine*, *157*, 2334–2341.

Pierson, H. M., Hayes, S. C., Gifford, E. V., Roget, N., Padilla, M., Bissett, R., et al. (2007). An examination of the motivational interviewing treatment integrity code. *Journal of Substance Abuse Treatment*, *32*(1), 11–17.

Prescott, P., Opheim, A., & Bortveit, T. (2002). The effect of workshops and training on counselling skills. *Journal of the Norwegian Psychological Association*, *5*, 426–431.

Rollnick, S., Kinnersley, P., & Butler, C. (2002). Context-bound communication skills training: Development of a new method. *Medical Education*, *36*(4), 377–383.

Rosengren, D. B., Baer, J. S., Hartzler, B., Dunn, C. W., & Wells, E. A. (2005). The Video Assessment of Simulated Encounters (VASE): Development and validation of a group-administered method for evaluating clinician skills in motivational interviewing. *Drug and Alcohol Dependence*, *79*, 321–330.

Rubak, S., Sandbaek, A., Lauritzen, T., Borch-Johnsen, K., & Christensen, B. (2006). An education and training course in motivational interviewing influence: GPs' professional behaviour. *British Journal of General Practice*, *56*, 429–436.

Schoener, E. P., Madeja, C. L., Henderson, M. J., Ondersma, S. J., & Janisse, J. J. (2006). Effects of motivational interviewing training on mental health therapist behavior. *Drug and Alcohol Dependence*, *82*, 269–275.

Thrasher, A. D., Golin, C. E., Earp, J. A., Tien, H., Porter, C., & Howie, L. (2005). Training general practitioners in behavior change counseling to improve asthma medication adherence. *Patient Education and Counseling*, *58*, 279–287.

Tober, G., Godfrey, C., Parrott, S., Copello, A., Farrin, A., Hodgson, R., et al. (2005). Setting standards for training and competence: The UK alcohol treatment trial. *Alcohol and Alcoholism*, *40*, 413–418.

Velasquez, M. M., Hecht, J., Quinn, V. P., Emmons, K. M., DiClemente, C. C., & Dolan-Mullen, P. (2000). Application of motivational interviewing to prenatal smoking cessation: Training and implementation issues. *Tobacco Control*, *9*(Suppl. 3), 36–40.

Welch, G., Rose, G., Hanson, D., Lekarcyk, J., Smith-Ossman, S., Gordon, T., et al. (2003). Changes in motivational interviewing skills code (misc) scores following motivational interviewing training for diabetes educators. *Diabetes*, *52*(Suppl. 1), A421.

APPENDIX B

A Topical Bibliography of Research on Motivational Interviewing

ALCOHOL/DRUG ABUSE

Adamson, S. J., & Sellman, J. D. (2001). Drinking goal selection and treatment outcome in out-patients with mild–moderate alcohol dependence. *Drug and Alcohol Review, 20,* 351–359.

Agostinelli, G., Brown, J. M., & Miller, W. R. (1995). Effects of normative feedback on consumption among heavy drinking college students. *Journal of Drug Education, 25,* 31–40.

Allsop, S., Saunders, B., Phillips, M., & Carr, A. (1997). A trial of relapse prevention with severely dependent male problem drinkers. *Addiction, 92,* 61–74.

Alwyn, T., John, B., Hodgson, R. J., & Phillips, C. J. (2004). The addition of a psychological intervention to a home detoxification programme. *Alcohol and Alcoholism, 39,* 536–541.

Anton, R. F., Moak, D. H., Latham, P., Waid, L. R., Myrick, H., Voronin, K., et al. (2005). Naltrexone combined with either cognitive behavioral or motivational enhancement therapy for alcohol dependence. *Journal of Clinical Psychopharmacology, 25,* 349–357.

Anton, R. F., O'Malley, S. S., Ciraulo, D. A., Couper, D., Donovan, D. M., Gastfriend, D. R., et al. (2006). Combined pharmacotherapies and behavioral interventions for alcohol dependence. The COMBINE study: A randomized controlled trial. *Journal of the American Medical Association, 295,* 2003–2017.

Aubrey, L. L. (1998). *Motivational interviewing with adolescents presenting for outpatient substance abuse treatment.* Unpublished doctoral dissertation, University of New Mexico.

Babor, T. F. (2004). Brief treatments for cannabis dependence: Findings from a randomized multisite trial. *Journal of Consulting and Clinical Psychology, 72,* 455–466.

Baer, J. S., Garrett, S. B., Beadnell, B., Wells, E. A., & Peterson, P. L. (in press). Brief motivational intervention with homeless adolescents: Evaluating effects on substance use and service utilization. *Psychology of Addictive Behaviors.*

Baer, J. S., Kivlahan, D. R., Blume, A. W., McKnight, P., & Marlatt, G. A. (2001). Brief intervention for heavy-drinking college students: 4-year follow-up and natural history. *American Journal of Public Health*, *91*, 1310–1316.

Baer, J. S., Marlatt, G. A., Kivlahan, D. R., Fromme, K., Larimer, M., & Williams, E. (1992). An experimental test of three methods of alcohol risk-reduction with young adults. *Journal of Consulting and Clinical Psychology*, *60*, 974–979.

Bailey, K. A., Baker, A. L., Webster, R. A., & Lewin, T. J. (2004). Pilot randomized controlled trial of a brief alcohol intervention group for adolescents. *Drug and Alcohol Review*, *23*(2), 157–166.

Baker, A., Boggs, T. G., & Lewin, T. J. (2001). Randomized controlled trial of brief cognitive-behavioural interventions among regular users of amphetamine. *Addiction*, *96*, 1279–1287.

Baker, A., Lee, N. K., Claire, M., Lewin, T. J., Grant, T., Pohlman, S., et al. (2005). Brief cognitive–behavioural interventions for regular amphetamine users: A step in the right direction. *Addiction*, *100*, 367–378.

Ball, S. A., Todd, M., Tennen, H., Armeli, S., Mohr, C., Affleck, G., et al. (2007). Brief motivational enhancement and coping skills interventions for heavy drinking. *Addictive Behaviors*, *32*, 1105–1118.

Barnett, N. P., Tevyaw, T. O., Fromme, K., Borsari, B., Carey, K. B., Corbin, W. R., et al. (2004). Brief alcohol interventions with mandated or adjudicated college students. *Alcoholism: Clinical and Experimental Research*, *77*, 49–59.

Battjes, R. J., Gordon, M. S., O'Grady, K. E., Kinlock, T. W., Katz, E. C., & Sears, E. A. (2004). Evaluation of a group-based substance abuse treatment program for adolescents. *Journal of Substance Abuse Treatment*, *27*, 123–134.

Bellack, A. S., Bennett, M. E., Gearon, J. S., Brown, C. H., & Yang, T. (2006). A randomized clinical trial of a new behavioral treatment for drug abuse in people with severe and persistent mental illness. *Archives of General Psychiatry*, *63*, 426–432.

Bennett, G. A., Edwards, S., & Bailey, J. (2002). Helping methadone patients who drink excessively to drink less: Short term outcomes of a pilot motivational intervention. *Journal of Substance Use*, *7*, 191–197.

Bernstein, J., Bernstein, E., Tassiopoulos, K., Heeren, T., Levenson, S., & Hingson, R. (2005). Brief motivational intervention at a clinic visit reduces cocaine and heroin use. *Drug and Alcohol Dependence*, *77*, 49–59.

Bien, T. H., Miller, W. R., & Boroughs, J. M. (1993). Motivational interviewing with alcohol outpatients. *Behavioural and Cognitive Psychotherapy*, *21*, 347–356.

Booth, R. E., Corsi, K. F., & Mikulich-Gilbertson, S. K. (2004). Factors associated with methadone maintenance treatment retention among street-recruited injection drug users. *Drug and Alcohol Dependence*, *74*, 177–185.

Borsari, B., & Carey, K. B. (2000). Effects of a brief motivational intervention with college student drinkers. *Journal of Consulting and Clinical Psychology*, *68*, 728–733.

Breslin, C., Li, S., Sdao-Jarvie, K., Tupker, E., & Ittig-Deland, V. (2002). Brief treatment for young substance abusers: A pilot study in an addiction treatment setting. *Psychology of Addictive Behaviors*, *16*, 10–16.

Brown, J. M., & Miller, W. R. (1993). Impact of motivational interviewing on participation and outcome in residential alcoholism treatment. *Psychology of Addictive Behaviors*, *7*, 211–218.

Brown, T. G., Dongier, M., Latimer, E., Legault, L., Seraganian, P., Kokin, M., et al. (2006). Group-delivered brief intervention versus standard care for mixed alcohol/other drug problems: A preliminary study. *Alcoholism Treatment Quarterly*, *24*, 23–40.

Budney, A. J., Higgins, S. T., Radonovich, K. J., & Novy, P. L. (2000). Adding voucher-based incentives to coping skills and motivational enhancement improves outcomes during treatment for marijuana dependence. *Journal of Consulting and Clinical Psychology*, *68*, 1051–1061.

Carroll, K. M., Ball, S. A., Nich, C., Martino, S., Frankforter, T. L., Farentinos, C., et al. (2006). Motivational interviewing to improve treatment engagement and outcome in individuals seeking treatment for substance abuse: A multisite effectiveness study. *Drug and Alcohol Dependence*, *81*, 301–312.

Carroll, K. M., Easton, C. J., Hunkele, K. A., Neavins, T. M., Sinha, R., Ford, H. L., et al. (2006). The use of contingency management and motivational/skills-building therapy to treat young adults with marijuana dependence. *Journal of Consulting and Clinical Psychology*, *74*, 955–966.

Carroll, K. M., Libby, B., Sheehan, J., & Hyland, N. (2001). Motivational interviewing to enhance treatment initiation in substance abusers: An effectiveness study. *American Journal on Addictions*, *10*, 335–339.

Cisler, R. A., Barrett, D. E., Zweben, A., & Berger, L. K. (2003). Integrating a brief motivational treatment in a private outpatient clinic: Client characteristics, utilization of services and preliminary outcomes. *Alcoholism Treatment Quarterly*, *21*(3), 1–21.

Collins, S. E., & Carey, K. B. (2005). Lack of effect for decisional balance as a brief motivational intervention for at-risk college drinkers. *Addictive Behaviors*, *30*, 1425–1430.

Connors, G. J., Walitzer, K. S., & Dermen, K. H. (2002). Preparing clients for alcoholism treatment: Effects on treatment participation and outcomes. *Journal of Consulting and Clinical Psychology*, *70*, 1161–1169.

Copello, A., Godfrey, C., Heather, N., Hodgson, R., Orford, J., Raistrick, D., et al. (2001). United Kingdom Alcohol Treatment Trial (UKATT): Hypotheses, design and methods. *Alcohol and Alcoholism*, *36*, 11–21.

D'Angelo, M. (2006). *A comparative study of motivational interviewing and traditional treatment approach on movement along stages of change, treatment completion, compliance with aftercare plan, and length of abstinence.* Unpublished doctoral dissertation.

Davidson, D., Gulliver, S. B., Longabaugh, R., Wirtz, P. W., & Swift, R. (2007). Building better cognitive-behavioral therapy: Is broad-spectrum treatment more effective than motivational-enhancement therapy for alcohol-dependent patients treated with naltrexone? *Journal of Studies on Alcohol and Drugs*, *68*, 238–247.

Davis, T. M., Baer, J. S., Saxon, A. J., & Kivlahan, D. R. (2003). Brief motivational feedback improves post-incarceration treatment contact among veterans with substance use disorders. *Drug and Alcohol Dependence*, *69*, 197–203.

Dennis, M., Godley, S. H., Diamond, G., Tims, F. M., Babor, T., Donaldson, J., et al. (2004). The Cannabis Youth Treatment (CYT) study: Main findings from two randomized trials. *Journal of Substance Abuse Treatment*, *27*, 197–213.

Dennis, M., Scott, C. K., & Funk, R. (2003). An experimental evaluation of recovery management checkups (RMC) for people with chronic substance use disorders. *Evaluation and Program Planning*, *26*, 339–352.

DeWildt, W., Schippers, G. M., Van den Brink, W., Potgeiter, A. S., Deckers, F., & Bets, D. (2002). Does psychosocial treatment enhance the efficacy of acamprosate in patients with alcohol problems? *Alcohol and Alcoholism*, *37*, 375–382.

Dunn, C. W., & Ries, R. (1997). Linking substance abuse services with general medical care: Integrated, brief interventions with hospitalized patients. *American Journal of Drug and Alcohol Abuse*, *23*, 1–13.

Dzialdowski, A., & London, M. (1999). A cognitive behavioural intervention in the context of methadone tapering treatment for opiate addiction: Two single cases. *Clinical Psychology and Psychotherapy*, *6*, 308–323.

Emmen, M. J., Schippers, G. M., Bleijenberg, G., & Wollersheim, H. (2005). Adding psychologist's intervention to physicians' advice to problem drinkers in the outpatient clinic. *Alcohol and Alcoholism*, *40*, 219–226.

Feldstein, S. W. (2007). *Motivational interviewing with late adolescent college underage drinkers: An investigation of therapeutic alliance.* Unpublished doctoral dissertation, University of New Mexico.

Floyd, R. L., Sobell, M., Velasquez, M. M., Ingersoll, K., Nettleman, M., Sobell, L., et al. (2007). Preventing alcohol-exposed pregnancies: A randomized controlled trial. *American Journal of Preventive Medicine, 32,* 1–10.

Foote, J., Deluca, A., Magura, S., Warner, A., Grand, A., Rosenblum, A., et al. (1999). A group motivational treatment for chemical dependency. *Journal of Substance Abuse Treatment, 17,* 181–192.

Gil, A. G., Wagner, E. F., & Tubman, J. G. (2004). Culturally sensitive substance abuse intervention for Hispanic and African American adolescents: Empirical examples from the Alcohol Treatment Targeting Adolescents in Need (ATTAIN) project. *Addiction, 99,* 140–150.

Gray, E., McCambridge, J., & Strang, J. (2005). The effectiveness of motivational interviewing delivered by youth workers in reducing drinking, cigarette and cannabis smoking among young people: Quasi-experimental pilot study. *Alcohol and Alcoholism, 40,* 535–539.

Grenard, J. L., Ames, S. L., Wiers, R. W., Thush, C., Stacy, A. W., & Sussman, S. (2007). Brief intervention for substance use among at-risk adolescents: A pilot study. *Journal of Adolescent Health, 40*(2), 188–191.

Handmaker, N. S., Hester, R. K., & Delaney, H. D. (1999). Videotaped training in alcohol counseling for obstetric care practitioners: A randomized controlled trial. *Obstetrics and Gynecology, 93,* 213–218.

Handmaker, N. S., Miller, W. R., & Manicke, M. (1999). Findings of a pilot study of motivational interviewing with pregnant drinkers. *Journal of Studies on Alcohol, 60,* 285–287.

Heather, N., Rollnick, S., Bell, A., & Richmond, R. (1996). Effects of brief counselling among heavy drinkers identified on general hospital wards. *Drug and Alcohol Review, 15,* 29–38.

Hester, R. K., Squires, D. D., & Delaney, H. D. (2005). The drinker's check-up: 12-month outcomes of a controlled clinical trial of a stand-alone software program for problem drinkers. *Journal of Substance Abuse, 28,* 159–169.

Hickman, M. E. (1999). *The effects of personal feedback on alcohol intake in dually diagnosed clients: An empirical study of William R. Miller's motivational enhancement therapy.* Unpublished doctoral dissertation.

Holder, H. D., Cisler, R. A., Longabaugh, R., Stout, R. L., Treno, A. J., & Zweben, A. (2000). Alcoholism treatment and medical care costs from Project MATCH. *Addiction, 95,* 999–1013.

Ingersoll, K., Floyd, L., Sobell, M., Velasquez, M. M., Baio, J., Carbonari, J., et al. (2003). Reducing the risk of alcohol-exposed pregnancies: A study of a motivational intervention in community settings. *Pediatrics, 111,* 1131–1135.

Ingersoll, K. S., Ceperich, S. D., Nettleman, M. D., Karanda, K., Brocksen, S., & Johnson, B. A. (2005). Reducing alcohol-exposed pregnancy risk in college women: Initial outcomes of a clinical trial of a motivational intervention. *Journal of Substance Abuse Treatment, 29,* 173–180.

John, U., Veltrup, C., Driessen, M., Wetterling, T., & Dilling, H. (2003). Motivational intervention: An individual counselling vs a group treatment approach for alcohol-dependent in-patients. *Alcohol and Alcoholism, 38*(3), 263–269.

Juarez, P., Walters, S. T., Daugherty, M., & Radi, C. (2006). A randomized trial of motivational interviewing and feedback with heavy drinking college students. *Journal of Drug Education, 36,* 233–246.

Kadden, R. M., Litt, M. D., Kabela-Cormier, E., & Petry, N. M. (2007). Abstinence rates following behavioral treatments for marijuana dependence. *Addictive Behaviors, 32,* 1220–1236.

Kahler, C. W., Read, J. P., Stuart, G., Ramsey, S. E., & McCrady, B. S. (2004). Motivational enhancement for 12-step involvement among patients undergoing alcohol detoxification. *Journal of Consulting and Clinical Psychology, 72*, 736–741.

Karno, M. P., & Longabaugh, R. (2004). What do we know? Process analysis and the search for a better understanding of Project MATCH's anger-by-treatment matching effect. *Journal of Studies on Alcohol, 65*, 501–512.

Kelly, A. B., Halford, W. K., & Young, R. M. (2000). Maritally distressed women with alcohol problems: The impact of a short-term alcohol-focused intervention on drinking behaviour and marital satisfaction. *Addiction, 95*, 1537–1549.

Knight, J. R., Sherritt, L., Van Hook, S., Gates, E. C., Levy, S., & Chang, G. (2005). Motivational interviewing for adolescent substance use: A pilot study. *Journal of Adolescent Health, 37*, 167–169.

Kranzler, H. R., Wesson, D. R., & Billot, L. (2004). Naltrexone depot for treatment of alcohol dependence: A multicenter, randomized, placebo-controlled clinical trial. *Alcoholism: Clinical and Experimental Research, 28*, 1051–1059.

Kuchipudi, V., Hobein, K., Fleckinger, A., & Iber, F. L. (1990). Failure of a 2-hour motivational intervention to alter recurrent drinking behavior in alcoholics with gastrointestinal disease. *Journal of Studies on Alcohol, 51*, 356–360.

Labrie, J. W., Lamb, T. F., Pedersen, E. R., & Quinlan, T. (2006). A group motivational interviewing intervention reduces drinking and alcohol-related consequences in adjudicated college students. *Journal of College Student Development, 47*, 267–280.

Labrie, J. W., Pederson, E. R., Lamb, T. F., & Quinlan, T. (2007). A campus-based motivational enhancement group intervention reduces problematic drinking in male college students. *Addictive Behaviors, 32*, 889–901.

Lapham, S. C., Chang, I. Y., & Gregory, C. (2000). Substance abuse intervention for health care workers: A preliminary report. *Journal of Behavioral Health Services and Research, 27*, 131–143.

Larimer, M. E., Turner, A. P., Anderson, B. K., Fader, J. S., Kilmer, J. R., Palmer, R. S., et al. (2001). Evaluating a brief alcohol intervention with fraternities. *Journal of Studies on Alcohol, 62*, 370–380.

Leontieva, L., Horn, K., Haque, A., Helmkamp, J., Ehrlich, P., & Williams, J. (2005). Readiness to change problematic drinking assessed in the emergency department as a predictor of change. *Journal of Clinical Care, 20*, 251–256.

Lincourt, P., Kuettel, T. J., & Bombardier, C. H. (2002). Motivational interviewing in a group setting with mandated clients: A pilot study. *Addictive Behaviors, 27*, 381–391.

Longabaugh, R., Wirtz, P. W., Zweben, A., & Stout, R. L. (1998). Network support for drinking, Alcoholics Anonymous and long-term matching effects. *Addiction, 93*, 1313–1333.

Longabaugh, R., Woolard, R. E., Nirenberg, T. D., Minugh, A. P., Becker, B., Clifford, P. R., et al. (2001). Evaluating the effects of a brief motivational intervention for injured drinkers in the emergency department. *Journal of Studies on Alcohol, 62*, 806–816.

Longshore, D., & Grills, C. (2000). Motivating illegal drug use recovery: Evidence for a culturally congruent intervention. *Journal of Black Psychology, 26*, 288–301.

Longshore, D., Grills, C., & Annon, K. (1999). Effects of a culturally congruent intervention on cognitive factors related to drug-use recovery. *Substance Use and Misuse, 34*, 1223–1241.

Maisto, S. A., Conigliaro, J., Mcneil, M., Kraemer, K., Conigliaro, R. L., & Kelley, M. E. (2001). Effects of two types of brief intervention and readiness to change on alcohol use in hazardous drinkers. *Journal of Studies on Alcohol, 62*, 605–614.

Marlatt, G. A., Baer, J. S., Kivlahan, D. R., Dimeff, L. A., Larimer, M. E., Quigley, L. A., et al. (1998). Screening and brief intervention for high-risk college student drinkers: Results from a 2-year follow-up assessment. *Journal of Consulting and Clinical Psychology, 66*, 604–615.

Marques, P. R., Voas, R. B., Tippetts, A. S., & Beirness, D. J. (1999). Behavioral monitoring of DUI offenders with the alcohol ignition interlock recorder. *Addiction, 94*(12), 1861–1870.

Marsden, J., Stilwell, G., Barlow, H., Boys, A., Taylor, C., Junt, N., et al. (2006). An evaluation of a brief motivational intervention among young Ecstasy and cocaine users: No effect on substance and alcohol use outcomes. *Addiction, 101*, 1014–1026.

Martin, G., Copeland, J., & Swift, W. (2005). The adolescent cannabis check-up: Feasibility of a brief intervention foryoung cannabis users. *Journal of Substance Abuse Treatment, 29*, 207–213.

McCambridge, J., & Strang, J. (2004). The efficacy of single-session motivational interviewing in reducing drug consumption and perceptions of drug-related risk and harm among young people: Results from a multi-site cluster randomized trial. *Addiction, 99*, 39–52.

McCambridge, J., & Strang, J. (2005). Deterioration over time in effect of motivational interviewing in reducing drug consumption and related risk among young people. *Addiction, 100*, 470–478.

McCambridge, J., Strang, J., Platts, S., & Witton, J. (2003). Cannabis use and the GP: Brief motivational intervention increases clinical enquiry by GPs in a pilot study. *British Journal of General Practice, 53*(493), 637–639.

Miller, W. R., Benefield, R. G., & Tonigan, J. S. (1993). Enhancing motivation for change in problem drinking: A controlled comparison of two therapist styles. *Journal of Consulting and Clinical Psychology, 61*, 455–461.

Miller, W. R., Sovereign, R. G., & Krege, B. (1988). Motivational interviewing with problem drinkers: II. The Drinker's Check-up as a preventive intervention. *Behavioural Psychotherapy, 16*, 251–268.

Miller, W. R., Toscova, R. T., Miller, J. H., & Sanchez, V. (2000). A theory-based motivational approach for reducing alcohol/drug problems in college. *Health Education and Behavior, 27*, 744–759.

Miller, W. R., Yahne, C. E., & Tonigan, J. S. (2003). Motivational interviewing in drug abuse services: A randomized trial. *Journal of Consulting and Clinical Psychology, 71*, 754–763.

Mitcheson, L., McCambridge, J., & Byrne, S. (2007). Pilot cluster-rendomized trial of adjunctive motivational interviewing to reduce crack cocaine use in clients on methadone maintenance. *European Addiction Research, 13*, 6–10.

Monti, P. M., Colby, S. M., Barnett, N. P., Spirito, A., Rohsenow, D. J., Myers, M., et al. (1999). Brief intervention for harm reduction with alcohol-positive older adolescents in a hospital emergency department. *Journal of Consulting and Clinical Psychology, 67*, 989–994.

Morgenstern, J., Irwin, T. W., Wainberg, M. L., Parsons, J. T., Muench, F., Bux, D. A., Jr., et al. (2007). A randomized controlled trial of goal choice interventions for alcohol use disorders among men who have sex with men. *Journal of Consulting and Clinical Psychology, 75*, 72–84.

Mullins, S. A., Suarez, M., Ondersma, S. J., & Page, M. C. (2004). The impact of motivational interviewing on substance abuse treatment retention: A randomized controlled trial of women involved with child welfare. *Journal of Substance Abuse Treatment, 27*(1), 521–558.

Murphy, J. G., Benson, T. A., Vuchinich, R. E., Deskins, M. M., Eakin, D., Flood, A. M., et al. (2004). A comparison of personalized feedback for college student drinkers delivered with and without a motivational interview. *Journal of Studies on Alcohol, 65*, 200–203.

Murphy, J. G., Duchnick, J. J., Vuchinich, R. E., Davison, J. W., Karg, R. S., Olson, A. M., et al. (2001). Relative efficacy of a brief motivational intervention for college student drinkers. *Psychology of Addictive Behaviors, 15*(4), 373–379.

Noonan, W. C. (2001). *Group motivational interviewing as an enhancement to outpatient alcohol treatment.* Unpublished doctoral dissertation, University of New Mexico.

Ondersma, S. J., Svikis, D. S., & Schuster, C. R. (2007). Computer-based motivational intervention for post-partum drug use: A randomized trial. *American Journal of Preventive Medicine, 32,* 231–238.

Peterson, P. L., Baer, J. S., Wells, E. A., Ginzler, J. A., & Garrett, S. B. (2006). Short-term effects of a brief motivational intervention to reduce alcohol and drug use among homeless adolescents. *Psychology of Addictive Behaviors, 20,* 254–264.

Project MATCH Research Group. (1997). Matching alcoholism treatments to client heterogeneity: Project MATCH posttreatment drinking outcomes. *Journal of Studies on Alcohol, 58,* 7–29.

Project MATCH Research Group. (1997). Project MATCH secondary a priori hypotheses. *Addiction, 92,* 1671–1698.

Project MATCH Research Group. (1998). Matching alcoholism treatments to client heterogeneity: Project MATCH three-year drinking outcomes. *Alcoholism: Clinical and Experimental Research, 22,* 1300–1311.

Project MATCH Research Group. (1998). Matching alcoholism treatments to client heterogeneity: Treatment main effects and matching effects on drinking during treatment. *Journal of Studies on Alcohol, 59,* 631–639.

Project MATCH Research Group. (1998). Matching patients with alcohol disorders to treatments: Clinical implications from Project MATCH. *Journal of Mental Health, 7,* 589–602.

Project MATCH Research Group. (1998). Therapist effects in three treatments for alcohol problems. *Psychotherapy Research, 8,* 455–474.

Reid, S. C., Teesson, M., Sannibale, C., Matsuda, M., & Haber, P. S. (2005). The efficacy of compliance therapy in pharmacotherapy for alcohol dependence: A randomized controlled trial. *Journal of Studies on Alcohol, 66,* 833–841.

Richmond, R., Heather, N., Kehoe, L, & Webster, I. (1995). Controlled evaluation of a general practice–based brief intervention for excessive drinking. *Addiction, 90,* 119–132.

Rohsenow, D. J., Monti, P. M., Martin, R. A., Colby, S. M., Myers, M. G., Gulliver, S. B., et al. (2004). Motivational enhancement and coping skills training for cocaine abusers: Effects on substance use outcomes. *Addiction, 99*(7), 862–874.

Rosenblum, A., Cleland, C., Magura, S., Mahmood, D., Kosanke, N., & Foote, J. (2005). Moderators of effects of motivational enhancements to cognitive behavioral therapy. *American Journal of Drug and Alcohol Abuse, 31,* 35–58.

Saitz, R., Palfai, T. P., Cheng, D. M., Horton, N. J., Freedner, N., Dukes, K., et al. (2007). Brief intervention for medical inpatients with unhealthy alcohol use: A randomized, controlled trial. *Annals of Internal Medicine, 146,* 167–176.

Sanchez, F. P. (2001). *A values-based intervention for alcohol abuse.* Unpublished doctoral dissertation, University of New Mexico.

Saunders, B., Wilkinson, C., & Phillips, M. (1995). The impact of a brief motivational intervention with opiate users attending a methadone programme. *Addiction, 90,* 415–424.

Schneider, R. J., Casey, J., & Kohn, R. (2000). Motivational versus confrontational interviewing: A comparison of substance abuse assessment practices at employee assistance programs. *Journal of Behavioral Health Services Research, 27,* 60–74.

Secades-Villa, R., Fernande-Hermida, J. R., & Arnaez-Montaraz, C. (2004). Motivational interviewing and treatment retention among drug user patients: A pilot study. *Substance Use and Misuse, 39*(9), 1369–1378.

Sellman, J. D., Sullivan, P. F., Dore, G. M., Adamson, S. J., & MacEwan, I. (2001). A randomized controlled trial of motivational enhancement therapy (MET) for mild to moderate alcohol dependence. *Journal of Studies on Alcohol*, *62*, 389–396.

Senft, R. A., Polen, M. R., Freeborn, D. K., & Hollis, J. F. (1997). Brief intervention in a primary care setting for hazardous drinkers. *American Journal of Preventive Medicine*, *13*, 464–470.

Sinha, R., Easton, C., Renee-Aubin, L., & Carroll, K. M. (2003). Engaging young probation-referred marijuana-abusing individuals in treatment: A pilot trial. *American Journal on Addictions*, *12*(4), 314–323.

Sobell, L. C., Sobell, M. B., Leo, G. I., Agrawal, S., Johnson-Young, L., & Cunningham, J. A. (2002). Promoting self-change with alcohol abusers: A community-level mail intervention based on natural recovery studies. *Alcoholism: Clinical and Experimental Research*, *26*, 936–948.

Spirito, A., Monti, P. M., Barnett, N. P., Colby, S. M., Sindelar, H., Rohsenow, D. J., et al. (2004). A randomized clinical trial of a brief motivational intervention for alcohol-pos itive adolescents treated in an emergency department. *Journal of Pediatrics*, *145*, 396–402.

Stein, L. A. R., & Lebeau-Craven, R. (2002). Motivational interviewing and relapse prevention for DWI: A pilot study. *Journal of Drug Issues*, *32*(4), 1051–1069.

Stein, L. A. R., Colby, S. M., Barnett, N. M., Monti, P. M., Golembeske, C., & Lebeau-Craven, R. (2006). Effects of motivational interviewing for incarcerated adolescents on driving under the influence after release. *American Journal of Addictions*, *15*(Suppl. 1), 50–57.

Stein, L. A. R., Colby, S. M., Barnett, N. P., Monti, P. M., Golembeske, C., Lebeau-Craven, R., et al. (2006). Enhancing substance abuse treatment engagement in incarcerated adolescents. *Psychological Services*, *3*, 25–34.

Stein, M. D., Anderson, B., Charuvastra, A., Maksad, J., & Friedman, P. D. (2002). A brief intervention for hazardous drinkers in a needle exchange program. *Journal of Substance Abuse Treatment*, *22*, 23–31.

Stephens, R. S., Roffman, R. A., & Curtin, L. (2000). Comparison of extended versus brief treatments for marijuana use. *Journal of Consulting and Clinical Psychology*, *68*, 898–908.

Stephens, R. S., Roffman, R. A., Fearer, S. A., Williams, C., & Burke, R. S. (2007). The marijuana check-up: Promoting change in ambivalent marijuana users. *Addiction*, *102*, 947–957.

Stockwell, T., & Gregson, A. (1986). Motivational interviewing with problem drinkers: Impact on attendance, drinking and outcome. *British Journal of Addiction*, *81*(5), 713.

Supplee, P. D. (2005). The importance of providing smoking relapse counseling during the postpartum hospitalization. *Journal of Obstetric, Gynecologic and Neonatal Nursing*, *34*, 703–712.

Thevos, A. K., Roberts, J. S., Thomas, S. E., & Randall, C. L. (2000). Cognitive behavioral therapy delays relapse in female socially phobic alcoholics. *Addictive Behaviors*, *25*(3), 333–345.

Thevos, A. K., Thomas, S. E., & Randall, C. L. (2001). Social support in alcohol dependence and social phobia: Treatment comparisons. *Research on Social Work Practice*, *11*(4), 458–472.

Walker, D. D., Roffman, R. A., Stephens, R. S., Wakana, K., Berghuis, J. P., & Kim, W. (2006). Motivational enhancement therapy for adolescent marijuana users: A preliminary randomized controlled trial. *Journal of Consulting and Clinical Psychology*, *74*, 628–632.

Walters, S. T., Bennett, M. E., & Miller, J. H. (2000). Reducing alcohol use in college students: A controlled trial of two brief interventions. *Journal of Drug Education*, *30*, 361–372.

White, H. R., Morgan, T. J., Pugh, L. A., Celinski, K., Labovie, E. W., & Pandina, R. J. (2006). Evaluating two brief substance-use interventions for mandated college students. *Journal of Studies on Alcohol*, *67*, 309–317.

Zywiak, W. H., Longabaugh, R., & Wirtz, P. W. (2002). Decomposing the relationships between pretreatment social network characteristics and alcohol treatment outcome. *Journal of Studies on Alcohol*, *63*(1), 114–121.

ASTHMA/COPD

Broers, S., Smets, E. M. A., Bindels, P., Evertsz, F. B., Calff, M., & DeHaes, H. (2005). Training general practitioners in behavior change counseling to improve asthma medication adherence. *Patient Education and Counseling*, *58*, 279–287.

de Blok, B. M., de Greef, M. H., ten Hacken, N. H., Sprenger, S. R., Postema, K., & Wempe, J. B. (2006). The effects of a lifestyle physical activity counseling program with feedback of a pedometer during pulmonary rehabilitation in patients with COPD: A pilot study. *Patient Education and Counseling*, *61*(1), 48–55.

Schmaling, K. B., Blume, A. W., & Afari, N. (2001). A randomized controlled pilot study of motivational interviewing to change attitudes about adherence to medications for asthma. *Journal of Clinical Psychology in Medical Settings*, *8*, 167–172.

BRAIN INJURY

Bell, K. R., Temkin, N. R., Esselman, P. C., Doctor, J. N., Bombardier, C. H., Fraser, R. T., et al. (2005). The effect of a scheduled telephone intervention on outcome after moderate to severe traumatic brain injury: A randomized trial. *Archives of Physical Medicine and Rehabilitation*, *86*, 851–856.

Bombardier, C. H., & Rimmele, C. T. (1999). Motivational interviewing to prevent alcohol abuse after traumatic brain injury: A case series. *Rehabilitation Psychology*, *44*, 52–67.

CARDIOVASCULAR HEALTH/HYPERTENSION

Beckie, T. M. (2006). A behavior change intervention for women in cardiac rehabilitation. *Journal of Cardiovascular Nursing*, *21*, 146–153.

Brodie, D. A., & Inoue, A. (2005). Motivational interviewing to promote physical activity for people with chronic heart failure. *Journal of Advanced Nursing*, *50*, 518–527.

McHugh, F., Lindsay, G. M., Hanlon, P., Hutton, I., Brown, M. R., Morrison, C., et al. (2001). Nurse-led shared care for patients on the waiting list for coronary artery bypass surgery: A randomised controlled trial. *Heart*, *86*(3), 317–323.

Ogedegbe, G., & Chaplin, W. (2005). Motivational interviewing improves systolic blood pressure in hypertensive African Americans [Abstract]. *American Journal of Hypertension*, *18*, A212.

Ogedegbe, G., Schoenthaler, A., Richardson, T., Lewis, L., Belue, R., Espinosa, E., et al. (2007). An RCT of the effect of motivational interviewing on medication adherence in hypertensive African Americans: Rationale and design. *Contemporary Clinical Trials*, *28*, 169–181.

Riegel, B., Dickson, W., Hoke, L., McMahon, J. P., Reis, B. F., & Sayers, S. (2006). A motivational counseling approach to improving heart failure self-care: Mechanisms of effectiveness. *Journal of Cardiovascular Nursing*, *21*, 232–241.

Scales, R. (1998). *Motivational interviewing and skills-based counseling in cardiac rehabilitation: The Cardiovascular Health Initiative and Lifestyle Education (CHILE) study.* Unpublished doctoral dissertation, University of New Mexico.

Scales, R., Lueker, R. D., Atterbom, H. A., Handmaker, N. S., & Jackson, K. A. (1997). Impact of motivational interviewing and skills-based counseling on outcomes in cardiac rehabilitation. *Journal of Cardiopulmonary Rehabilitation*, *17*, 328.

Watkins, C. L., Anton, M. F., Deans, C. F., Dickinson, H. A., Jack, C. I., Lightbody, C. E., et al. (2007). Motivational interviewing early after acute stroke: A randomized, controlled trial. *Stroke*, *38*, 1004–1009.

Woollard, J., Beilin, L., Lord, T., Puddey, I., MacAdam, D., & Rouse, I. (1995). A controlled trial of nurse counselling on lifestyle change for hypertensives treated in general practice: Preliminary results. *Clinical and Experimental Pharmacology and Physiology*, *22*, 466–468.

Woollard, J., Burke, V., & Beilin, L. J. (2003). Effects of general practice–based nurse-counselling on ambulatory blood pressure and antihypertensive drug prescription in patients at increased risk of cardiovascular disease. *Journal of Human Hypertension*, *17*, 689–695.

Woollard, J., Burke, V., Beilin, L. J., Verheijden, M., & Bulsara, M. K. (2003). Effects of a general practice–based intervention on diet, body mass index and blood lipids in patients at cardiovascular risk. *Journal of Cardiovascular Risk*, *10*, 31–40.

DENTISTRY

Skaret, E., Weinstein, P., Kvale, G., & Raadal, M. (2003). An intervention program to reduce dental avoidance behaviour among adolescents: A pilot study. *European Journal of Paediatric Dentistry*, *4*, 191–196.

Weinstein, P., Harrison, R., & Benton, T. (2004). Motivating parents to prevent caries in their young children: One-year findings. *Journal of the American Dental Association*, *135*(6), 731–738.

Weinstein, P., Harrison, R., & Benton, T. (2006). Motivating mothers to prevent caries: Confirming the beneficial effect of counseling. *Journal of the American Dental Association*, *137*, 789–793.

DIABETES

Channon, S., Smith, V. J., & Gregory, J. W. (2003). A pilot study of motivational interviewing in adolescents with diabetes. *Archives of Disease in Childhood*, *88*(8), 680–683.

Clark, M., & Hampson, S. E. (2001). Implementing a psychological intervention to improve lifestyle self-management in patients with type 2 diabetes. *Patient Education and Counseling*, *42*, 247–256.

Hokanson, J. M., Anderson, R. L., Hennrikus, D. J., Lando, H. A., & Kendall, D. M. (2006). Integrated tobacco cessation counseling in a diabetes self-management training program: A randomized trial of diabetes and reduction of tobacco. *Diabetes Educator*, *32*, 562–570.

Rubak, S., Sandbaek, A., Lauritzen, T., Borch-Johnsen, K., & Christensen, B. (in press). Effect of the motivational interview on measures of quality care in people with screen detected type 2 diabetes: A one-year follow-up of a RCT. *British Journal of General Practice*.

Rubak, S., Sandbaek, A., Lauritzen, T., Borch-Johnsen, K., & Christensen, B. (in press). A RCT study: Effect of "motivational interviewing" on beliefs and behaviour among patients with type 2 diabetes detected by screening. *Scandinavian Journal of Public Health*.

Smith, D. E., Heckemeyer, C. M., Kratt, P. P., & Mason, D. A. (1997). Motivational interviewing to improve adherence to a behavioral weight-control program for older obese women with NIDDM: A pilot study. *Diabetes Care*, *20*, 52–54.

Trigwell, P., Grant, P. J., & House, A. (1997). Motivation and glycemic control in diabetes mellitus. *Journal of Psychosomatic Research*, *43*, 307–315.

Viner, R. M., Christie, D., Taylor, V., & Hey, S. (2003). Motivational/solution-focused intervention improves HbA_{1c} in adolescents with type 1 diabetes: A pilot study. *Diabetic Medicine*, *20*(9), 739–742.

West, D. S., DiLillo, V., Bursac, Z., Gore, S. A., & Greene, P. G. (2007). Motivational interviewing improves weight loss with type 2 diabetes. *Diabetes Care*, *30*, 1081–1087.

DIET/LIPIDS

Berg-Smith, S. M., Stevens, V. J., Brown, K. M., Van Horn, L., Gernhofer, N., Peters, E., et al. (1999). A brief motivational intervention to improve dietary adherence in adolescents. *Health Education Research*, *14*, 399–410.

Bowen, D., Ehret, C., Pedersen, M., Snetselaar, L., Johnson, M., Tinker, L., et al. (2002). Results of an adjunct dietary intervention program in the women's health initiative. *Journal of the American Dietetic Association*, *102*(11), 1631–1637.

Bowen, D. J., Beresford, S. A. A., Vu, T., Fend, Z. D., Tinker, L., Hart, A., et al. (2004). Baseline data and design for a randomized intervention study of dietary change in religious organizations. *Preventive Medicine*, *39*, 602–611.

Brug, J., Spikmans, F., Aartsen, C., Breedveld, B., Bes, R., & Fereira, I. (2007). Training dietitians in basic motivational interviewing skills results in changes in their counseling style and in lower saturated fat intakes in their patients. *Journal of Nutrition Education and Behavior*, *39*, 8–12.

Fuemmeler, B. F., Masse, L. C., Yaroch, A. L., Resnicow, K., Campbell, M. K., Carr, C., et al. (2006). Psychosocial mediation of fruit and vegetable consumption in the Body and Soul effectiveness trial. *Health Psychology*, *25*, 474–483.

Mhurchu, C. N., Margetts, B. M., & Speller, V. (1998). Randomized clinical trial comparing the effectiveness of two dietary interventions with hyperlipidaemia. *Clinical Science*, *95*, 479–487.

Resnicow, K., Campbell, M. K., Carr, C., McCarty, F., Wang, T., Periasamy, S., et al. (2004). Body and soul: A dietary intervention conducted through African-American churches. *American Journal of Preventive Medicine*, *27*, 97–105.

Resnicow, K., Coleman-Wallace, D., Jackson, A., Digirolamo, A., Odom, E., Wang, T., et al. (2000). Dietary change through black churches: Baseline results and program description of the Eat for Life trial. *Journal of Cancer Education*, *15*, 156–163.

Resnicow, K., Jackson, A., Blissett, D., Wang, T., McCarty, F., Rahotep, S., et al. (2005). Results of the Healthy Body Healthy Spirit trial. *Health Psychology*, *24*, 339–348.

Resnicow, K., Jackson, A., Wang, T., De, A. K., McCarty, F., Dudley, W. N., et al. (2001). A motivational interviewing intervention to increase fruit and vegetable intake through Black churches: Results of the Eat for Life trial. *American Journal of Public Health*, *91*, 1686–1693.

Resnicow, K., Taylor, R., Baskin, M., & McCarty, F. (2005). Results of Go Girls: A weight control program for overweight African-American adolescent females. *Obesity Research*, *13*, 1739–1748.

Richards, A., Kettelmann, K. K., & Ren, C. R. (2006). Motivating 18- to 24-year-olds to increase their fruit and vegetable consumption. *Journal of the American Dietetic Association*, *106*, 1405–1411.

Wen, D. B., Ehret, C., Pedersen, M., Snetselaar, L., Johnson, M., Tinker, L., et al. (2002). Abstract results of an adjunct dietary intervention program in the Women's Health Initiative. *Journal of the American Dietetic Association, 102*(11), 1631–1637.
West, D. S., DiLillo, V., Bursac, Z., Gore, S. A., & Greene, P. G. (2007). Motivational interviewing improves weight loss with type 2 diabetes. *Diabetes Care, 30*, 1081–1087.
Woollard, J., Burke, V., Beilin, L. J., Verheijden, M., & Bulsara, M. K. (2003). Effects of a general practice–based intervention on diet, body mass index and blood lipids in patients at cardiovascular risk. *Journal of Cardiovascular Risk, 10*, 31–40.

DOMESTIC VIOLENCE

Kennerley, R. J. (2000). *The ability of a motivational pre-group session to enhance readiness for change in men who have engaged in domestic violence.* Unpublished doctoral dissertation.
Kistenmacher, B. R. (2000). *Motivational interviewing as a mechanism for change in men who batter: A randomized controlled trial.* Unpublished doctoral dissertation, University of Oregon.

DUAL DIAGNOSIS (SUBSTANCE USE DISORDER AND MENTAL ILLNESS)

Baker, A., Bucci, S., Lewin, T., Kay-Lambkin, F., Constable, P. M., & Carr, V. J. (2006). Cognitive-behavioral therapy for substance use disorders in people with psychotic disorders: Randomized clinical trial. *British Journal of Psychiatry, 188*, 439–444.
Baker, A., Lewin, T., Reichler, H., Clancy, R., Carr, V., Garrett, R., et al. (2002). Evaluation of a motivational interview for substance use within psychiatric in-patient services. *Addiction, 97*(10), 1329–1337.
Barrowclough, C., Haddock, G., Tarrier, N., Lewis, S. W., Moring, J., O'Brien, R., et al. (2001). Randomized controlled trial of motivational interviewing, cognitive behavior therapy, and family intervention for patients with comorbid schizophrenia and substance use disorders. *American Journal of Psychiatry, 158*, 1706–1713.
Brown, R. A., Ramsey, S. E., Strong, D. R., Myers, M. G., Kahler, C. W., Lejuez, C. W., et al. (2003). Effects of motivational interviewing on smoking cessation in adolescents with psychiatric disorders. *Tobacco Control, 12*(Suppl. 4), 3–10.
Carey, K. B., Carey, M. P., Maisto, S. A., & Purnine, D. M. (2002). The feasibility of enhancing psychiatric outpatients' readiness to change their substance use. *Psychiatric Services, 53*, 602–608.
Daley, D. C., Salloum, I. M., Zuckoff, A., Kirisci, L., & Thase, M. E. (1998). Increasing treatment adherence among outpatients with depression and cocaine dependence: Results of a pilot study. *American Journal of Psychiatry, 155*, 1611–1613.
Daley, D. C., & Zuckoff, A. (1998). Improving compliance with the initial outpatient session among discharged inpatient dual diagnosis clients. *Social Work, 43*, 470–473.
Graeber, D. A., Moyers, T. B., Griffith, G., Guajardo, E., & Tonigan, J. S. (2003). A pilot study comparing motivational interviewing and an educational intervention in patients with schizophrenia and alcohol use disorders. *Community Mental Health Journal, 39*, 189–202.
Haddock, G., Barrowclough, C., Tarrier, N., Moring, J., O'Brien, R., Schofield, N., et al. (2003). Cognitive-behavioural therapy and motivational intervention for schizophrenia

and substance misuse: 18-month outcomes of a randomized controlled trial. *British Journal of Psychiatry, 183*, 377–378.

Hulse, G. K., & Tait, R. J. (2002). Six-month outcomes associated with a brief alcohol intervention for adult in-patients with psychiatric disorders. *Addiction, 21*, 105–112.

Hulse, G. K., & Tait, R. J. (2003). Five-year outcomes of a brief alcohol intervention for adult in-patients with psychiatric disorders. *Addiction, 98*, 1061–1068.

Kavanagh, D. J., Young, R., White, A., Saunders, J. B., Wallis, J., Shockley, N., et al. (2004). A brief motivational intervention for substance misuse in recent-onset psychosis. *Drug and Alcohol Review, 23*, 151–155.

Kreman, R., Yates, B. C., Agrawal, S., Fiandt, K., Briner, W., & Shurmur, S. (2006). The effects of motivational interviewing on physiological outcomes. *Applied Nursing Research, 19*, 167–170.

Martino, S., Carroll, K. M., Nich, C., & Rounsaville, B. J. (2006). A randomized controlled pilot study of motivational interviewing for patients with psychotic and drug use disorders. *Addiction, 101*, 1479–1492.

Martino, S., Carroll, K. M., O'Malley, S. S., & Rounsaville, B. J. (2000). Motivational interviewing with psychiatrically ill substance abusing patients. *American Journal on Addictions, 9*, 88–91.

Santa Ana, E. J. (2005). *Efficacy of group motivational interviewing (GMI) for psychiatric inpatients with chemical dependence.* Unpublished doctoral dissertation.

Swanson, A. J., Pantalon, M. V., & Cohen, K. R. (1999). Motivational interviewing and treatment adherence among psychiatric and dually-diagnosed patients. *Journal of Nervous and Mental Disease, 187*, 630–635.

Tapert, S. F., Colby, S. M., Barnett, N. P., Spirito, A., Rohsenow, D. J., Myers, M. G., et al. (2003). Depressed mood, gender, and problem drinking in youth. *Journal of Child and Adolescent Substance Abuse, 12*(4), 55–68.

Zuckoff, A., Shear, K., Frank, E., Daley, D. C., Seligman, K., & Silowash, R. (2006). Treating complicated grief and substance use disorders: A pilot study. *Journal of Substance Abuse Treatment, 30*, 205–211.

EATING DISORDERS/OBESITY

Dunn, E. C., Neighbors, C., & Larimer, M. (2006). Motivational enhancement therapy and self-help treatment for binge eaters. *Psychology of Addictive Behaviors, 20*, 44–52.

Feld, R., Woodside, D. B., Kaplan, A. S., Olmsted, M. P., & Carter, J. C. (2001). Pretreatment motivational enhancement therapy for eating disorders: A pilot study. *International Journal of Eating Disorders, 29*, 393–400.

Long, C. G., & Hollin, C. R. (1995). Assessment and management of eating disordered patients who over-exercise: A four-year follow-up of six single case studies. *Journal of Mental Health, 4*, 309–316.

Pung, M. A., Niemeier, H. M., Cirona, A. C., Barrera, A. Z., & Craighead, L. W. (2004). Motivational interviewing in the reduction of risk factors for eating disorders: A pilot study. *International Journal of Eating Disorders, 35*(4), 396–397.

Smith, D. E., Heckemeyer, C. M., Kratt, P. P., & Mason, D. A. (1997). Motivational interviewing to improve adherence to a behavioral weight-control program for older obese women with NIDDM: A pilot study. *Diabetes Care, 20*, 52–54.

Treasure, J. L., Katzman, M., Schmidt, U., Troop, N., Todd, G., & De Silva, P. (1999). Engagement and outcome in the treatment of bulimia nervosa: First phase of a sequential design comparing motivation enhancement therapy and cognitive behavioural therapy. *Behaviour Research and Therapy, 37*, 405–418.

EMERGENCY DEPARTMENT/TRAUMA/INJURY PREVENTION

Dunn, C., Droesch, R. M., Johnston, B. D., & Rivara, F. P. (2004). Motivational interviewing with injured adolescents in the emergency department: In-session predictors of change. *Behavioural and Cognitive Psychotherapy, 32*(1), 113–116.

Johnston, B. D., Rivara, F. P., & Droesch, R. M. (2002). Behavior change counseling in the emergency department to reduce injury risk: A randomized, controlled trial. *Pediatrics, 110*, 267–274.

Schermer, C. R., Moyers, T. B., Miller, W. R., & Bloomfield, L. A. (2006). Trauma center brief interventions for alcohol disorders decrease subsequent driving under the influence arrests. *Journal of Trauma, 60*, 29–34.

Zatzick, D., Roy-Byrne, P., Russo, J., Rivara, F., Droesch, R., Wagner, A., et al. (2004). A randomized effectiveness trial of stepped collaborative care for acutely injured trauma survivors. *Archives of General Psychiatry, 61*(5), 498–506.

FAMILY/RELATIONSHIPS

Cordova, J. V., Scott, R. G., Dorian, M., Mirgain, S., Yeager, D., & Groot, A. (2005). The marriage check-up: An indicated preventive intervention for treatment-avoidant couples at risk for marital deterioration. *Behavior Therapy, 36*, 301–309.

Kelly, A. B., Halford, W. K., & Young, R. M. (2000). Maritally distressed women with alcohol problems: The impact of a short-term alcohol-focused intervention on drinking behaviour and marital satisfaction. *Addiction, 95*, 1537–1549.

Naar-King, S., Wright, K., Parsons, J. T., Frey, M., Templin, T., Lam, P., et al. (2006). Healthy choices: Motivational enhancement therapy for health risk behaviors in HIV-positive youth. *AIDS Education and Prevention, 18*, 1–11.

O'Leary, C. C. (2001). *The early childhood family check-up: A brief intervention for at-risk families with preschool-aged children.* Unpublished doctoral dissertation.

Rao, S. O. (1999). *The short-term impact of the family check-up: A brief motivational intervention for at-risk families.* Unpublished doctoral dissertation.

Slavert, J. D., Stein, L. A. R., Klein, J. L., Colby, S. M., Barnett, N. P., & Monti, P. M. (2005). Piloting the family check-up with incarcerated adolescents and their parents. *Psychological Services, 2*, 123–132.

Uebelacker, L. A., Hecht, J., & Miller, I. W. (2006). The family check-up: A pilot study of a brief intervention to improve family functioning in adults. *Family Process, 45*, 223–236.

GAMBLING

Hodgins, D. C., Currie, S. R., & el-Guebaly, N. (2001). Motivational enhancement and self-help treatments for problem gambling. *Journal of Consulting and Clinical Psychology, 69*, 50–57.

Hodgins, D. C., Currie, S., el-Guebaly, N., & Peden, N. (2004). Brief motivational treatment for problem gambling: A 24-month follow-up. *Psychology of Addictive Behaviors, 18*, 293–296.

Kuentzel, J. G., Henderson, M. J., Zambo, J. J., Stine, S. M., & Schuster, C. R. (2003). Motivational interviewing and fluoxetine for pathological gambling disorder: A single case study. *North American Journal of Psychology, 5*(2), 229–248.

Wulfert, E., Blanchard, E. B., Freidenberg, B. M., & Martell, R. S. (2006). Retaining pathological gamblers in cognitive behavior therapy through motivational enhancement: A pilot study. *Behavior Modification, 30*, 315–340.

HEALTH PROMOTION/EXERCISE/FITNESS

Bennett, J. A., Lyons, K. S., Winters-Stone, K., Nail, L. M., & Scherer, J. (2007). Motivational interviewing to increase physical activity in long-term cancer survivors: A randomized controlled trial. *Nursing Research, 56*, 18–27.

Brodie, D. A., & Inoue, A. (2005). Motivational interviewing to promote physical activity for people with chronic heart failure. *Journal of Advanced Nursing, 50*, 518–527.

Butterworth, S., Linden, A., McClay, W., & Leo, M. C. (2006). Effect of motivational interviewing–based health coaching on employees' physical and mental health status. *Journal of Occupational Health Psychology, 11*, 358–365.

Elliot, D. L., Goldberg, L., Duncan, T. E., Kuehl, K. S., & Moe, E. L. (2004). The PHLAME firefighters' study: Feasibility and findings. *American Journal of Health Behavior, 28*, 13–23.

Elliot, D. L., Goldberg, L., Kuehl, K. S., Moe, E. L., Breger, R. K., & Pickering, M. A. (2007). The PHLAME (Promoting Healthy Lifestyles: Alternative Models' Effects) firefighter study: Outcomes of two models of behavior change. *Journal of Occupational and Environmental Medicine, 49*, 204–213.

Harland, J., White, M., Drinkwater, C., Chinn, D., Farr, L., & Howel, D. (1999). The Newcastle Exercise Project: A randomised controlled trial of methods, to promote physical activity in primary care. *British Medical Journal, 319*, 828–832.

Hillsdon, M., Thorogood, N., White, I., & Foster, C. (2002). Advising people to take more exercise is ineffective: A randomised controlled trial of physical activity promotion in primary care. *International Journal of Epidemiology, 31*, 808–815.

Hudec, J. C. (2000). *Individual counseling to promote physical activity.* Unpublished doctoral dissertation.

Kolt, G. S., Oliver, M., Schofield, G. M., Kerse, N., Garrett, N., & Latham, N. K. (2006). An overview and process evaluation of Telewalk: A telephone-based counseling intervention to encourage walking in older adults. *Health Promotion International, 21*, 201–208.

Ludman, E. J., Curry, S. J., Meyer, D., & Taplin, S. H. (1999). Implementation of outreach telephone counseling to promote mammography participation. *Health Education and Behavior, 26*, 689–702.

Moe, E. L., Elliot, D. L., Goldberg, L., Kuehl, K. S., Stevens, V. J., Breger, R. K. R., et al. (2002). Promoting healthy lifestyles: Alternative models' effects (PHLAME). *Health Education Research, 17*(5), 586–596.

Thevos, A. K., Kaona, F. A. D., Siajunza, M. T., & Quick, R. E. (2000). Adoption of safe water behaviors in Zambia: Comparing educational and motivational approaches. *Education for Health* (joint issue with the *Annual of Behavioral Sciences and Medical Education*), *13*, 366–376.

Thevos, A. K., Olsen, S. J., Rangel, J. M., Kaona, F. A. D., Tembo, M., & Quick, R. E. (2002–2003). Social marketing and motivational interviewing as community interventions for safe water behaviors: Follow-up surveys in Zambia. *International Quarterly of Community Health Education, 21*, 51–65.

Thevos, A. K., Quick, R. E., & Yanjuli, V. (2000). Motivational interviewing enhances the adoption of water disinfection practices in Zambia. *Health Promotion International, 15*, 207–214.

Valanis, B., Whitlock, E. E., Mullooly, J., Vogt, T., Smith, S., Chen, C. H., et al. (2003).

Screening rarely screened women: Time-to-service and 24-month outcomes of tailored interventions. *Preventive Medicine*, *37*(5), 442–450.

Valanis, B. G., Glasgow, R. E., Mullooly, J., Vogt, T. M., Whitlock, E. P., Boles, S. M., et al. (2002). Screening HMO women overdue for both mammograms and Pap tests. *Preventive Medicine*, *34*, 40–50.

van Vilsteren, M. C., de Greef, M. H. G., & Huisman, R. M. (2005). The effects of a low-to-moderate intensity pre-conditioning exercise programme linked with exercise counselling for sedentary haemodialysis patients in the Netherlands: A randomized clinical trial. *Nephrology Dialysis Transplantation*, *20*, 141–146.

Wilhelm, S. L., Stepans, M. B., Hertzog, M., Rodehorst, T. K., & Gardner, P. (2006). Motivational interviewing to promote sustained breastfeeding. *Journal of Obstetrical, Gynecological, and Neonatal Nursing*, *35*, 340–348.

HIV/AIDS

Aharonovich, E., Hartzenbuehler, M. L., Johnston, B., O'Leary, A., Morgenstern, J., Wainberg, M. L., et al. (2006). A low-cost, sustainable intervention for drinking reduction in the HIV primary care settings. *AIDS Care: Psychological and Socio-Medical Aspects of AIDS/HIV*, *18*, 561–568.

Baker, A., Heather, N., Wodak, A., Dixon, J., & Holt, P. (1993). Evaluation of a cognitive behavioral intervention for HIV prevention among injecting drug users. *AIDS*, *7*, 247–256.

Carey, M. P., Braaten, L. S., Maisto, S. A., Gleason, J. R., Forsyth, A. D., Durant, L. E., et al. (2000). Using information, motivational enhancement, and skills training to reduce the risk of HIV infection for low-income urban women: A second randomized clinical trial. *Health Psychology*, *19*, 3–11.

Carey, M. P., Maisto, S. A., Kalichman, S. C., Forsyth, A. D., Wright, E. M., & Johnson, B. T. (1997). Using information, motivational enhancement, and skill training to reduce the risk of HIV infection for low-income urban women: A second randomized clinical trial. *Journal of Consulting and Clinical Psychology*, *65*, 531–541.

Dilorio, C., Resnicow, K., McDonnell, M., Soet, J., McCarty, F., & Yeager, K. (2003). Using motivational interviewing to promote adherence to antiretroviral medications: A pilot study. *Journal of the Association of Nurses in AIDS Care*, *14*(2), 52–62.

Golin, C. E., Earp, J. L., Tien, H. C., Stewart, P., Porter, C., & Howie, L. (2006). A 2-arm, randomized, controlled trial of a motivational interviewing–based intervention to improve adherence to antiretroviral therapy (ART) among patients failing or initiating ART. *Journal of Acquired Immune Deficiency Syndrome*, *42*, 42–51.

Kalichman, S. C., Cherry, C., & Browne-Sperling, F. (1999). Effectiveness of a video-based motivational skills–building HIV risk-reduction intervention for inner-city African American men. *Journal of Consulting and Clinical Psychology*, *67*, 959–966.

Knight, J. R., Sherritt, L., Van Hook, S., Gates, E. C., Levy, S., & Chang, G. (2005). Motivational interviewing for adolescent substance use: A pilot study. *Journal of Adolescent Health*, *37*, 167–169.

Koblin, B., Chesney, M., Coates, T., & Team, E. S. (2004). Effects of a behavioural intervention to reduce acquisition of HIV infection among men who have sex with men: The EXPLORE randomised controlled study. *Lancet*, *364*, 41–50.

Naar-King, S., Wright, K., Parsons, J. T., Frey, M., Templin, T., Lam, P., et al. (2006). Healthy choices: Motivational enhancement therapy for health risk behaviors in HIV-positive youth. *AIDS Education and Prevention*, *18*, 1–11.

Parsons, J. T., Rosof, E., Punzalan, J. C., & DiMaria, I. (2005). Integration of motivational interviewing and cognitive behavioral therapy to improve HIV medication adherence and reduce substance use among HIV-positive men and women: Results of a pilot project. *AIDS Patient Care and STDs*, *19*, 31–39.

Patterson, T. L., Semple, S. J., Fraga, M., Bucardo, J., Davila-Fraga, W., & Strathdee, S. A. (2005). An HIV-prevention intervention for sex workers in Tijuana, Mexico: A pilot study. *Hispanic Journal of Behavioral Sciences*, *27*, 82–100.

Picciano, J. F., Roffman, R. A., Kalichman, S. C., Rutledge, S. E., & Berghuis, J. P. (2001). A telephone based brief intervention using motivational enhancement to facilitate HIV risk reduction among MSM: A pilot study. *AIDS and Behavior*, *5*, 251–262.

Robles, R. R., Reyes, J. C., Colon, H. M., Sahai, H., Marrero, C. A., Matos, T. D., et al. (2004). Effects of combined counseling and case management to reduce HIV risk behaviors among Hispanic drug injectors in Puerto Rico: A randomized controlled trial. *Journal of Substance Abuse Treatment*, *27*, 145–152.

Samet, J. H., Horton, N. J., Meli, S., Dukes, K., Tripps, T., Sullivan, L., et al. (2005). A randomized controlled trial to enhance antiretroviral therapy adherence in patients with a history of alcohol problems. *Antiviral Therapy*, *10*, 83–93.

Stein, M. D., Anderson, B., Charuvastra, A., Maksad, J., & Friedman, P. D. (2002). A brief intervention for hazardous drinkers in a needle exchange program. *Journal of Substance Abuse Treatment*, *22*, 23–31.

Thrasher, A. D., Golin, C. E., Earp, J. A. L., Tien, H., Porter, C., & Howie, L. (2006). Motivational interviewing to support antiretroviral therapy adherence: The role of quality counseling. *Patient Education and Counseling*, *62*, 64–71.

MEDICAL ADHERENCE

Aliotta, S. L., Vlasnik, J. J., & Delor, B. (2004). Enhancing adherence to long-term medical therapy: A new approach to assessing and treating patients. *Advances in Therapy*, *21*, 214–231.

Bennett, J. A., Perrin, N. A., & Hanson, G. (2005). Healthy aging demonstration project: Nurse coaching for behavior change in older adults. *Research in Nursing and Health*, *28*, 187–197.

Berger, B. A., Liang, H., & Hudmon, K. S. (2005). Evaluation of software-based telephone counseling to enhance medication persistency among patients with multiple sclerosis. *Journal of the American Pharmacists Association*, *45*, 466–472.

Broers, S., Smets, E. M. A., Bindels, P., Evertsz, F. B., Calff, M., & DeHaes, H. (2005). Training general practitioners in behavior change counseling to improve asthma medication adherence. *Patient Education and Counseling*, *58*, 279–287.

Hayward, P., Chan, N., Kemp, R., & Youle, S. (1995). Medication self-management: A preliminary report on an intervention to improve medication compliance. *Journal of Mental Health*, *4*, 511–518.

Kreman, R., Yates, B. C., Agrawal, S., Fiandt, K., Briner, W., & Shurmur, S. (2006). The effects of motivational interviewing on physiological outcomes. *Applied Nursing Research*, *19*, 167–170.

Robles, R. R., Reyes, J. C., Colon, H. M., Sahai, H., Marrero, C. A., Matos, T. D., et al. (2004). Effects of combined counseling and case management to reduce HIV risk behaviors among Hispanic drug injectors in Puerto Rico: A randomized controlled trial. *Journal of Substance Abuse Treatment*, *27*, 145–152.

Rose, J., & Walker, S. (2000). Working with a man who has Prader–Willi syndrome and his support staff using motivational principles. *Behavioural and Cognitive Psychotherapy*, *28*, 293–302.

MENTAL HEALTH

Arkowitz, H., Westra, H. A., Miller, W. R., & Rollnick, S. (Eds.). (2008). *Motivational interviewing in the treatment of psychological problems*. New York: Guilford Press.

Humphress, H., Igel, V., Lamont, A., Tanner, M., Morgan, J., & Schmidt, U. (2002). The effect of a brief motivational intervention on community psychiatric patients' attitudes to their care, motivation to change, compliance and outcome: A case control study. *Journal of Mental Health*, *11*, 155–166.

Kemp, R., Hayward, P., Applewhaite, G., Everitt, B., & David, A. (1996). Compliance therapy in psychotic patients: Randomised controlled trial. *British Medical Journal*, *312*, 345–349.

Kemp, R., Kirov, G., Everitt, B., Hayward, P., & David, A. (1998). Randomised controlled trial of compliance therapy: 18-month follow-up. *British Journal of Psychiatry*, *172*, 413–419.

Ludman, E., Simon, F., Tutty, S., & Von Korff, M. (2007). A randomized trial of telephone psychotherapy and pharmacotherapy support for depression: Continuation and durability of effects. *Journal of Consulting and Clinical Psychology*, *75*, 257–266.

Murphy, R. T., & Cameron, R. P. (2002). Development of a group treatment for enhancing motivation to change PTSD syndrome. *Cognitive and Behavioral Practice*, *9*, 308–316.

Simon, G., Ludman, E. J., Tutty, S., Operskalski, B., & Von Korff, M. (2004). Telephone psychotherapy and telephone care management for primary care patients starting antidepressant treatment: A randomized controlled trial. *Journal of the American Medical Association*, *292*, 935–942.

Westra, H. A., & Phoenix, E. (2003). Motivational enhancement therapy in two cases of anxiety disorder: New responses to treatment refractoriness. *Clinical Case Studies*, *2*(4), 306–322.

OFFENDERS

Harper, R., & Hardy, S. (2000). An evaluation of motivational interviewing as a method of intervention with clients in a probation setting. *British Journal of Social Work*, *30*, 393–400.

Mann, R., & Rollnick, S. (1996). Motivational interviewing with a sex offender who believed he was innocent. *Behavioural and Cognitive Psychotherapy*, *24*, 127–134.

Marques, P. R., Voas, R. B., Tippetts, A. S., & Beirness, D. J. (1999). Behavioral monitoring of DUI offenders with the alcohol ignition interlock recorder. *Addiction*, *94*(12), 1861–1870.

Sinha, R., Easton, C., Renee-Aubin, L., & Carroll, K. M. (2003). Engaging young probation-referred marijuana-abusing individuals in treatment: A pilot trial. *American Journal on Addictions*, *12*(4), 314–323.

Slavert, J. D., Stein, L. A. R., Klein, J. L., Colby, S. M., Barnett, N. P., & Monti, P. M. (2005). Piloting the family check-up with incarcerated adolescents and their parents. *Psychological Services*, *2*, 123–132.

Stein, L. A. R., Colby, S. M., Barnett, N. P., Monti, P. M., Golembeske, C., Lebeau-Craven, R., et al. (2006). Enhancing substance abuse treatment engagement in incarcerated adolescents. *Psychological Services*, *3*, 25–34.

Stein, L. A. R., & Lebeau-Craven, R. (2002). Motivational interviewing and relapse prevention for DWI: A pilot study. *Journal of Drug Issues*, *32*(4), 1051–1069.

PAIN

Ang, D., Kesavalu, R., Lydon, J. R., Lane, K. A., & Bigatti, S. (in press). Exercise-based motivational interviewing for female patients with fibromyalgia: A case series. *Clinical Rheumatology, 26.*

SEXUAL BEHAVIOR

Kiene, S. M., & Barta, W. D. (2006). A brief individualized computer-delivered sexual risk reduction intervention increases HIV/AIDS preventive behavior. *Journal of Adolescent Health, 39,* 404–410.

Mann, R., & Rollnick, S. (1996). Motivational interviewing with a sex offender who believed he was innocent. *Behavioural and Cognitive Psychotherapy, 24,* 127–134.

Orzack, M. H., Voluse, A. C., Wolf, D., & Hennen, J. (2006). An ongoing study of group treatment for men involved in problematic Internet-enabled sexual behavior. *Cyberpsychology and Behavior, 9,* 348–360.

Peterson, R., Albright, J., Garrett, J. M., & Curtis, K. M. (2007). Pregnancy and STD prevention counseling using an adaptation of motivational interviewing: A randomized controlled trial. *Perspectives on Sexual Reproductive Health, 39*(1), 21–28.

Yahne, C. E., Miller, W. R., Irvin-Vitela, L., & Tonigan, J. S. (2002). Magdalena pilot project: Motivational outreach to substance abusing women street sex workers. *Journal of Substance Abuse Treatment, 23*(1), 49–53.

SPEECH/VOCAL THERAPY

Behrman, A. (2006). Facilitating behavioral change in voice therapy: The relevance of motivational interviewing. *American Journal of Speech–Language Pathology, 15,* 215–225.

TOBACCO

Ahluwalia, J. S., Nollen, N., Kaur, H., James, A. S., Mayo, M. S., & Resnicow, K. (2007). Pathway to health: Cluster-randomized trial to increase fruit and vegetable consumption among smokers in public housing. *Health Psychology, 26,* 214–221.

Ahluwalia, J. S., Okuyemi, K., Nollen, N., Choi, W. S., Kaur, H., Pulvers, K., et al. (2006). The effects of nicotine gum and counseling among African American light smokers: A 2 × 2 factorial design. *Addiction, 101,* 833–891.

Baker, A., Richmond, R., Haile, M., Lewin, T. J., Carr, V. J., Taylor, R. L., et al. (2006). A randomized controlled trial of a smoking cessation intervention among people with a psychotic disorder. *American Journal of Psychiatry, 163,* 1934–1942.

Boardman, T., Catley, D., Grobe, J. E., Little, T. D., & Ahluwalia, J. S. (2006). Using motivational interviewing with smokers: Do therapist behaviors relate to engagement and therapeutic alliance? *Journal of Substance Abuse Treatment, 31,* 329–339.

Borelli, B., Novak, S., Hecht, J., Emmons, K., Papandonatos, G., & Abrams, D. (2005). Home health care nurses as a new channel for smoking cessation treatment: Outcomes from Project CARES (Community-Nurse Assisted Research and Education on Smoking). *Preventive Medicine, 41,* 815–821.

Brown, R. A., Ramsey, S. E., Strong, D. R., Myers, M. G., Kahler, C. W., Lejuez, C. W., et al. (2003). Effects of motivational interviewing on smoking cessation in adolescents with psychiatric disorders. *Tobacco Control, 12*(Suppl. 4), 3–10.

Butler, C. C., Rollnick, S., Cohen, D., Bachmann, M., Russell, I., & Stott, N. (1999). Motivational consulting versus brief advice for smokers in general practice: A randomized trial. *British Journal of General Practice, 49*, 611–616.

Chan, S. S., Lam, T. H., Salili, F., Leung, G. M., Wong, D. C., Botelho, R. J., et al. (2005). A randomized controlled trial of an individualized motivational intervention on smoking cessation for parents of sick children: A pilot study. *Applied Nursing Research, 18*, 178–181.

Cigrang, J. A., Severson, H. H., & Peterson, A. L. (2002). Pilot evaluation of a population-based health intervention for reducing use of smokeless tobacco. *Nicotine and Tobacco Research, 4*(1), 127–131.

Colby, S. M., Barnett, N. M., Monti, P. M., Rohsenow, D. J., Weissman, K., Spirito, A., et al. (1998). Brief motivational interviewing in a hospital setting for adolescent smoking: A preliminary study. *Journal of Consulting and Clinical Psychology, 66*, 574–578.

Colby, S. M., Monti, P. M., & Tevyaw, T. O. (2005). Brief motivational intervention for adolescent smokers in medical settings. *Addictive Behaviors, 30*, 865–874.

Curry, S. J., Ludman, E. J., Graham, E., Stout, J., Grothaus, L., & Lozano, P. (2003). Pediatric-based smoking cessation intervention for low-income women: A randomized trial. *Archives of Pediatrics and Adolescent Medicine, 157*, 295–302.

Emmons, K. M., Hammond, S. K., Fava, J. L., Velicer, W. F., Evans, J. L., & Monroe, A. D. (2001). A randomized trial to reduce passive smoke exposure in low-income households with young children. *American Academy of Pediatrics, 108*, 18–24.

Ershoff, D. H., Quinn, V. P., Boyd, N. R., Stern, J., Gregory, M., & Wirtschafter, D. (1999). The Kaiser Permanente prenatal smoking-cessation trial: When more isn't better, what is enough? *American Journal of Preventive Medicine, 17*, 161–168.

Gariti, P., Alterman, A., Mulvaney, F., Mechanic, K., Dhopesh, V., Yu, E., et al. (2002). Nicotine intervention during detoxification and treatment for other substance use. *American Journal of Drug and Alcohol Abuse, 28*, 673–681.

George, T. P., Ziedonis, D. M., Feingold, A., Pepper, W. T., Satterburg, C. A., Winkel, J., et al. (2000). Nicotine transdermal patch and atypical antipsychotic medications for smoking cessation in schizophrenia. *American Journal of Psychiatry, 157*, 1835–1842.

Glasgow, R. E., Whitlock, E. E., Eakin, E. G., & Lichtenstein, E. (2000). A brief smoking cessation intervention for women in low-income planned parenthood clinics. *American Journal of Public Health, 90*, 786–789.

Haug, N. A., Svikis, D. S., & DiClemente, C. C. (2004). Motivational enhancement therapy for nicotine dependence in methadone-maintained pregnant women. *Psychology of Addictive Behaviors, 18*, 289–292.

Helstrom, A., Hutchinson, K., & Bryan, A. (2007). Motivational enhancement therapy for high-risk adolescent smokers. *Addictive Behaviors, 32*, 2404–2410.

Hokanson, J. M., Anderson, R. L., Hennrikus, D. J., Lando, H. A., & Kendall, D. M. (2006). Integrated tobacco cessation counseling in a diabetes self-management training program: A randomized trial of diabetes and reduction of tobacco. *Diabetes Educator, 32*, 562–570.

Hollis, J. F., Polen, M. R., Whitlock, E. P., Lichtenstein, E., Mullooly, J., Velicer, W. F., et al. (2005). Teen Reach: Outcomes from a randomized controlled trial of a tobacco reduction program for teens seen in primary medical care. *Pediatrics, 115*, 981–989.

Horn, K., Dino, G., Hamilton, C., & Noerachmanto, N. (2007). Efficacy of an emergency department–based teenage smoking intervention. *Prevention of Chronic Disease, 4*, A08.

Kelley, A. B., & Lapworth, K. (2006). The HYP program: Targeted motivational interviewing for adolescent violations of school tobacco policy. *Preventive Medicine, 43*, 466–471.

Luna, L. (2005). *The effectiveness of motivational enhancement therapy on smoking cessation in college students.* Unpublished doctoral dissertation.

Nollen, N. L., Mayo, M. S., Sanderson Cox, L., Okuyemi, K. S., Choi, W. S., Kaur, H., et al. (2006). Predictors of quitting among African American light smokers enrolled in a randomized, placebo-controlled trial. *Journal of General Internal Medicine, 21*, 590–595.

Okuyemi, K., Cox, L. S., Nollen, N. L., Snow, T. M., Kaur, H., Choi, W. S., et al. (2007). Baseline characteristics and recruitment strategies in a randomized clinical trial of African-American light smokers. *American Journal of Health Promotion, 21*, 183–189.

Okuyemi, K. S., James, A. S., Mayo, M. S., Nollen, N., Catley, D., Choi, W. S., et al. (2007). Pathways to health: A cluster randomized trial of nicotine gum and motivational interviewing for smoking cessation in low-income housing. *Health Education and Behavior, 34*, 43–54.

Okuyemi, K. S., Thomas, J. L., Hall, S., Nollen, N. L., Richter, K. P., Jeffries, S. K., et al. (2006). Smoking cessation in homeless populations: A pilot clinical trial. *Nicotine and Tobacco Research, 8*, 689–699.

Pbert, L., Osganian, S. K., Gorak, D., Druker, S., Reed, G., O'Neill, K. M., et al. (2006). A school nurse–delivered adolescent smoking cessation intervention: A randomized controlled trial. *Preventive Medicine, 43*, 312–320.

Persson, L. G., & Hjalmarson, A. (2006). Smoking cessation in patients with diabetes mellitus: Results from a controlled study of an intervention programme in primary healthcare in Sweden. *Scandinavian Journal of Primary Health Care, 24*(2), 75–80.

Richter, K. P., McCool, R. M., Catley, D., Hall, M., & Ahluwalia, J. S. (2005). Dual pharmacotherapy and motivational interviewing for tobacco dependence among drug treatment patients. *Journal of Addictive Diseases, 24*, 79–90.

Rigotti, N. A., Park, E. R., Regan, S., Chang, Y., Perry, K., Loudin, B., et al. (2006). Efficacy of telephone counseling for pregnant smokers: A randomized controlled trial. *Obstetrics and Gynecology, 108*, 83–92.

Rohsenow, D. J., Martin, R. A., Monti, P. M., Abrams, D. B., Colby, S. M., & Sirota, A. D. (2004). Brief advice versus motivational interviewing for smoking with alcoholics in treatment [Abstract]. *Alcoholism: Clinical and Experimental Research, 28*, 76A.

Smith, S. S., Jorenby, D. E., Fiore, M. C., Anderson, J. E., Mielke, M. M., Beach, K. E., et al. (2001). Strike while the iron is hot: Can stepped-care treatments resurrect relapsing smokers? *Journal of Consulting and Clinical Psychology, 69*, 429–439.

Soria, R., Legido, A. Escolano, C., Yeste, A. L., & Montoya, J. (2006). A randomised controlled trial of motivational interviewing for smoking cessation. *British Journal of General Practice, 56*, 768–774.

Steinberg, M. L., Ziedonis, D. M., Krejci, J. A., & Brandon, T. H. (2004). Motivational interviewing with personalized feedback: A brief intervention for motivating smokers with schizophrenia to seek treatment for tobacco dependence. *Journal of Consulting and Clinical Psychology, 72*(4), 723–728.

Stotts, A. L., DeLaune, K. A., Schmitz, J. M., & Grabowski, J. (2004). Impact of a motivational intervention on mechanisms of change in low-income pregnant smokers. *Addictive Behaviors, 29*, 1649–1657.

Stotts, A. L., DiClemente, C. C., & Dolan-Mullen, P. (2002). One-to-one: A motivational intervention for resistant pregnant smokers. *Addictive Behaviors, 27*, 275–292.

Supplee, P. D. (2005). The importance of providing smoking relapse counseling during the postpartum hospitalization. *Journal of Obstetric, Gynecologic and Neonatal Nursing, 34*, 703–712.

Tappin, D. M., Lumsden, M. A., Gilmour, W. H., Crawford, F., McIntyre, D., Stone, D. H., et al. (2005). Randomised controlled trial of home based motivational interviewing by midwives to help pregnant smokers quit or cut down. *British Medical Journal, 331*, 373–377.

Thyrian, J. R., Freyer-Adam, J., Hannover, W., Roske, K., Mentzel, F., Kufeld, C., et al. (2007). Adherence to the principles of motivational interviewing, clients' characteristics and behavior outcome in a smoking cessation and relapse prevention trial in women postpartum. *Addictive Behaviors, 32*, 2297–2303.

Thyrian, J. R., Hanover, W., Grempler, J., Roske, K., John, U., & Hapke, U. (2006). An intervention to support postpartum women to quit smoking or remain smoke-free. *Journal of Midwifery and Women's Health, 51*, 45–50.

Town, G. I., Fraser, P., Graham, S., McSweeney, W., Brockway, K., & Kirk, R. (2000). Establishment of a smoking cessation programme in primary and secondary care in Canterbury. *New Zealand Medical Journal, 113*, 117–119.

Valanis, B., Lichtenstein, E., Mullooly, J. P., Labuhn, K., Brody, K., Severson, H. H., et al. (2001). Maternal smoking cessation and relapse prevention during health care visits. *American Journal of Preventive Medicine, 20*(1), 1–8.

Wakefield, M., Oliver, I., Whitford, H., & Rosenfeld, E. (2004). Motivational interviewing as a smoking cessation intervention for patients with cancer: Randomized controlled trial. *Nursing Research, 53*, 396–405.

Winickoff, J. P., Hillis, V. J., Palfrey, J. S., Perrin, J. M., & Rigotti, N. A. (2003). A smoking cessation intervention for parents of children who are hospitalized for respiratory illness: The stop tobacco outreach program. *Pediatrics, 111*(1), 140–145.

Woodruff, S. I., Conway, T. L., Edwards, C. C., Elliott, S. P., & Crittenden, J. (2006). Evaluation of an Internet virtual world chat room for adolescent smoking cessation. *Addictive Behaviors, 32*, 1769–1786.

Ziedonis, D., Harris, P., Brandt, P., Trudeau, K., George, T., Rao, S., et al. (1997). Motivational enhancement therapy and nicotine replacement improve smoking cessation outcomes for smokers with schizophrenia or depression. *Addiction, 92*, 633.

Index

Ability, 37
Adherence
  MI outcome studies, 199
  promoting, 98–107
Agendas, setting, 53–55, 151–152
Alcohol studies, 183–191
Ambivalence
  discussion of, 34–35
  resolving, 116–120
  working through with reflective listening, 83
Asking
  closed questions, 44–45, 46–47
  combining listening with, 75–76
  as a communication skill, 19
  may be a "roadblock" to listening, 69
  in motivational interviewing, 51, 53–55
  open questions, 45–46, 47–49
  practical suggestions for, 56–64
  the question–answer trap, 49–50
  relationship to communication styles, 21, 22
  routine assessments and, 50–51
  skillful practice in, 46–48
  using with other communication skills, 112–114, 115
Aspirations for patient behavior change (ABC), 146–148
Assessments, 167–168
Asthma studies, 191
Attentiveness, 141–142
Autonomy. *See* Patient autonomy

Behavior change. *See* Health behavior change
Behavior-change consultations. *See* Consultations
Brain injury studies, 191
"Bubble sheet" strategy, 54–55

Cardiac rehabilitation services, 164–170
Cardiovascular health studies, 191–192
Case examples
  cardiac rehabilitation services, 131–138, 164–170
  general medicine, 121–125
  HIV/AIDS services, 162–164
  public health promotion, 170, 172
  safe sex promotion, 126–130
Change talk
  guiding patients through, 41–42
  how the forms fit together, 40–41

Change talk (*continued*)
  kinds of, 36–40
  listening for, 35–41
  practical suggestions for questions to elicit, 56–64
  reflecting, 80–82
Chunk–check–chunk strategy
  examples, 99–100, 101–102
  mindset in, 96–97
  overview of, 94–95
Closed questions
  excessive reliance on, 46–47
  overview of, 44–45
Collaboration, 6
Commitment
  language indicating, 37, 39
  language to use when assessing, 118
  listening for, 117–120
Communication skills
  common use of, 20
  overview of, 19–20
  relationship to communication styles, 21
  used with communication styles, 21–28
  using flexibly within consultations, 29–30
  using in combinations, 112–116
  See also individual skills
Communication styles
  directing, 14–15, 17–18
  following, 14
  guiding, 15
  learning to shift between, 173–174
  mixing and matching, 15–17
  overview of, 12–14
  relationship of communication skills to, 21
  use of communication skills with, 21–28
  using flexibly within consultations, 29–30
  See also individual styles
Consultations
  asking questions in, 46–48
  case examples. *See* Case examples
  general guideline for, 175–176
  maintaining flexibility within, 29–30
  reviewing for self-improvement, 154–155
  when agendas differ, 150–153
  when to use listening in, 67
  where directing seems essential, 152–153
Control, letting go of, 142
COPD studies, 191

DARN
  eliciting change talk and, 40–41, 57–58
  meaning of term, 38
Denial, 144
Dentistry studies, 192
Desire, 36, 37
Diabetes studies, 192–193
Diet studies, 193–194
Directing style
  compared to other communication styles, 12–14
  dangers of falling into, 148
  discussion of, 14–15
  examples of, 22–25
  overuse of, 17–18
  relationship of communication skills to, 21, 22–25
  situations when necessary, 152–153
  using with other communication styles, 15–17
Domestic violence studies, 194
Drinking water safety, 170, 172
Drug abuse studies, 183–191
Dual-diagnosis studies, 194–195

Eating disorders studies, 195
Elicit–provide–elicit strategy (EPE)
  discussion of, 95–98
  example for promoting adherence, 100–101
  example for sharing test results, 102–104
Empowerment, 10
Equipoise, 147–148

Evocation, 6–7
Exercise studies, 197–198
Eye contact, 68

Family/relationships studies, 196
Feedback, 178–179
Fitness studies, 197–198
Following style
  compared to other communication styles, 12–14
  discussion of, 14
  relationship of communication skills to, 21, 25–27
  using with other communication styles, 15–17

Gambling studies, 196–197
Groups
  guidelines for guiding in, 171–172
  for patient education, 168–169
Guided participation, 155
Guiding style
  becoming skillful at, 174
  compared to other communication styles, 12–14
  getting used to, 140–141
  in groups, 171–172
  integrating with directing, 153
  and the issue of responsibility, 142–143
  judging the effectiveness of, 119–120
  looking ahead and letting go of control, 142
  motivational interviewing and, 18–19, 33
  overcoming obstacles, 143–153
  and the patient's struggles with change, 144–145
  practicing in everyday life, 155–156
  and the practitioner's feelings, 145–150
  relationship of communication skills to, 21, 27–28
  staying in the present, 141–142
  using with other communication styles, 15–17
  watching the relationship and, 141
  when agendas differ, 150–153

Health behavior change
  asking about commitment to, 62–63
  asking about pros and cons of, 61–62
  aspirations for, 146–148
  current need for, 3–4
  the myth of the unmotivated patient, 5–6
  the patient's struggles with, 144–145
  removing service system barriers to, 158–164
  taking steps statements, 37, 39–40
  See also Change talk; Readiness-to-change
Health care information. *See* Information
Health care providers. *See* Practitioners
Health care systems
  barriers to motivational interviewing in, 157–158
  removing barriers to change, 158–164
Health promotion studies, 197–198
HIV/AIDS
  MI outcome studies, 197–198
  providing an innovation in services, 162–164
  safe sex promotion, 126–130
Hypertension studies, 191–192
Hypothetical questions/language, 63–64

Information
  delivering with care, 90
  eliciting the patient to interpret, 104–105
  including positive messages with, 89–90
  overloading patients with, 149
  understanding the patient's needs and wishes for, 90

Information exchange
  guidelines for improving, 88–90
  using the directing style in, 90–91
  See also Informing
Information gathering
  with closed questions, 44–45
  following style and, 25–26
  with open questions, 45–46
Informing
  asking permission for, 91–92
  chunk–check–chunk strategy, 94–95, 96–97
  common difficulties experienced in, 86–88
  as a communication skill, 19–20
  directing with care, 90–91
  eliciting the patient to interpret information, 104–105
  elicit–provide–elicit strategy, 95–98
  examples, 98–107
  offering options, 93
  pitfalls of the righting reflex, 98
  to promote adherence, 99–101
  providing hope and, 105–107
  relationship to communication styles, 21, 22
  sharing test results, 101–104
  situations used in, 86
  talking about what others do, 93–94
  using with other communication skills, 112–113, 114–116
  working within a relationship, 88–90
  See also Information exchange
Injury prevention studies, 196
Internal dilemmas, acting out of, 8

Key questions, 62–63

Lipid studies, 193–194
Listening
  in combination with asking, 75–76
  for commitment, 117–120
  as a communication skill, 19
  concerns about, 76–77
  facilitative responses, 70
  following style and, 14
  in motivational interviewing, 77–85, 111–112
  opening steps in, 68–69
  to patients, 9
  practicing in everyday life, 155
  questions may be "roadblocks" to, 69
  by reflecting, 70–74
  relationship to communication styles, 21, 22
  silence and, 69–70
  summaries, 74–75
  using with other communication skills, 113–116
  value of, 65–66
  when to use, 66–67
  See also Reflective listening

Making the Patient Your Partner (Gordon & Edwards), 9
Medical adherence
  outcome studies, 199
  promoting, 99–101
Medical consultations. *See* Consultations
Mental health studies, 200
MI. *See* Motivational interviewing
MI "spirit," 6–7
Motivation
  the myth of the unmotivated patient, 5–6
  understanding in patients, 9
Motivational interviewing (MI)
  aids to learning, 178–179
  can seem familiar, 11–12
  case examples. *See* Case examples
  guiding principles, 7–10
  guiding style and, 18–19, 33
  implementing, 164–172
  the myth of the unmotivated patient, 5–6
  origin and development of, 4–5
  overview of, 111–112
  phases in learning, 173–175
  refining one's skills in, 174–175
  service system barriers to, 157–158

"spirit" of, 6–7
trainers in, 180
Motivational Interviewing Network of Trainers (MINT), 180

Need, 37, 38–39
Nonverbal cues, good listeners and, 68

Obesity studies, 195
Offender studies, 200
Open questions
examples of, 48–49
features and advantages of, 45–46
in skillful asking, 47–48

Pain studies, 201
Parenting, communication styles and, 16
Patient education groups, 168–169
Patients
aspirations for behavior change, 146–148
autonomy, 7
communicating with when upset, 26–27
guiding through change talk, 41–42
information and, 90, 104–105, 149
listening to, 9
motivation and, 5–6
obtaining permission from, 91–92
persuading too hard, 148–149
struggles with change, 144–145
Permission, obtaining from patients, 91–92
Persuasion–resistance trap, 148–149
Practitioners
aspirations for patient behavior change, 146–148
descending into directing, 148
feedback and, 178–179
following the patients and getting lost, 149
how feelings affect guiding, 145–150
notions of rescuing patients, 149
overloading patients with information, 149
overuse of the directing style, 17–18
persuading patients too hard, 148–149
protecting one's health, 154
pursuing problems and weaknesses, 150
reviewing consultations for self-improvement, 154–155
Premature focus, 53–54
Public health, 170, 172

Quantity–frequency investigation, 50
Question–answer trap, 49–50
Questions
closed, 44–45, 46–47
combining with listening, 75–76
may be "roadblocks" to listening, 69
open, 45–46, 47–49
See also Asking

Rating scales, 58–59, 60
Readiness-to-change, assessing, 60–61
Reasons, 37–38
Referrals, encouraging, 27–28
Reflecting, 70–74
Reflective listening
choosing what to reflect, 78–79
overview of, 70–74
reflecting change talk, 80–82
reflecting resistance, 79–80
summaries, 83–85
and working through ambivalence, 83
Resistance
persuasion–resistance trap, 148–149
reflecting, 79–80
Responsibility, 142–143
Righting reflex, 7–9, 98
Routine assessments, 50–51, 52

RULE principles
  overview of, 7–10
  using, 56–57
Rulers, 58–59, 60

Safe sex promotion, 126–130
Scaffolding, 155
Sexual behavior studies, 201
Silence, in listening, 69–70
Speech/vocal therapy studies, 201
Substance abuse service, 158–162
Summaries, 74–75, 83–85

Teaching, communication styles and, 16
Team meetings, 166–167
Test results, sharing, 101–104
Tobacco studies, 201–204
Trainers, 180
Trauma studies, 196
Treatment requests, 26

Unmotivated patients, myth of, 5–6

Zambia, 170